MEDICAL MANAGEMENT OF
TYPE 2 DIABETES

FIFTH EDITION

Charles F. Burant, MD, PhD, Editor

American Diabetes Association.

Cure • Care • Commitment®

Director, Book Publishing, John Fedor; *Associate Director, Professional Books, and Editor,* Christine B. Charlip; *Copy Editor,* Wendy M. Martin; *Associate Director, Book Production,* Peggy M. Rote; *Composition,* Circle Graphics; *Cover Design,* Koncept, Inc.; *Printer,* Port City Press

Printed in the United States of America
1 3 5 7 9 10 8 6 4 2

The suggestions and information contained in this publication are generally consistent with the *Clinical Practice Recommendations* and other policies of the American Diabetes Association, but they do not represent the policy or position of the Association or any of its boards or committees. Reasonable steps have been taken to ensure the accuracy of the information presented. However, the American Diabetes Association cannot ensure the safety or efficacy of any product or service described in this publication. Individuals are advised to consult a physician or other appropriate health care professional before undertaking any diet or exercise program or taking any medication referred to in this publication. Professionals must use and apply their own professional judgment, experience, and training and should not rely solely on the information contained in this publication before prescribing any diet, exercise, or medication. The American Diabetes Association—its officers, directors, employees, volunteers, and members—assumes no responsibility or liability for personal or other injury, loss, or damage that may result from the suggestions or information in this publication.

⊗ The paper in this publication meets the requirements of the ANSI Standard Z39.48-1992 (permanence of paper).

ADA titles may be purchased for business or promotional use or for special sales. To purchase this book in large quantities, or for custom editions of this book with your logo, contact Lee Romano Sequeira, Special Sales & Promotions, at the address below, or at LRomano@diabetes.org or call 703-299-2046.

American Diabetes Association
1701 North Beauregard Street
Alexandria, Virginia 22311

Library of Congress Cataloging-in-Publication Data

Medical management of type 2 diabetes / Charles F. Burant, editor.—5th ed.
    p. ; cm.
  Includes bibliographical references and index.
  ISBN 1-58040-189-9 (pbk. : alk. paper)
    1. Non-insulin-dependent diabetes. I. Title: Medical management of type two diabetes.
II. Burant, Charles F. III. American Diabetes Association.
  [DNLM: 1. Diabetes Mellitus, Type II. WK 810 M48791 2004]
  RC662.18.M43 2004
  616.4'62—dc22

                                                            2004052836

MEDICAL MANAGEMENT OF

TYPE 2

DIABETES

FIFTH EDITION

Contents

A Word About This Guide ix

Contributors to the Fifth Edition xi

Acknowledgments xiii

Diagnosis and Classification 1

Highlights 2

Types of Diabetes Mellitus and Other Categories
of Glucose Intolerance 3
Type 1 Diabetes 5
Type 2 Diabetes 6
The Metabolic Syndrome 7
Other Specific Types of Diabetes 7
Pre-Diabetes 8
Gestational Diabetes Mellitus 10

Screening for Diabetes Mellitus 10

Diagnostic Criteria for Diabetes Mellitus 11
Type 1 and Type 2 Diabetes 11
Pre-Diabetes 12
Gestational Diabetes Mellitus 12

Evaluation and Classification of Patients Before Treatment 13

Pathogenesis 17

Highlights 18

Genetic and Environmental Factors 19

Insulin Resistance 20
   Sites of Insulin Resistance 20
   Mechanisms of Insulin Resistance 20

The Fat Cell as an Endocrine Organ 22

Defects in Insulin Secretion 22
   Factors Modulating Insulin Secretion 23
   Physiological Consequences of Defective Insulin Secretion 23

Conclusion 23

Tools of Therapy 27

Highlights 29

Therapeutic Objectives and Plan 33

Nutrition 36
   Body Weight 37
   Protein 40
   Fat 41
   Carbohydrate 43
   Sugar and Fat Substitutes 44
   Vitamins and Minerals 45
   Alcohol 46

Exercise 48
   Benefits of Exercise 48
   Type and Duration of Exercise 49
   Preexercise Evaluation 50

Pharmacologic Intervention for Glycemia 52
   Available Agents 52
   Selecting an Agent to Begin Treatment 61
   Primary and Secondary Failure of Treatments 63
   Starting Insulin Therapy 63
   Long-Term Combinations of Oral Agents with Insulin 67
   Adjusting Insulin Dosage in Long-Term Type 2 Diabetes 68

Assessment of Treatment Efficacy 71
   Office Methods 72
   Patient Monitoring 74

Special Therapeutic Situations 79

Highlights 80

Pregnancy 83

Diabetes in Youth 85
   Differentiating Type 1 and Type 2 Diabetes in Youth 85
   Screening for Type 2 Diabetes in Youth 85
   Treating Type 2 Diabetes in Youth 85

Hospitalized, Surgical, and Critically Ill Patients 88

Hyperosmolar Hyperglycemic State 91
   Pathophysiology 91
   Therapy 92
   Identification and Treatment of Precipitating Causes 94
   Risks of Aggressive Treatment 94

Detection and Treatment of Chronic Complications 95

Highlights 97

Rationale for Optimizing Glycemic Control in Type 2 Diabetes 100

Accelerated Macrovascular Disease 101
   Diabetes as a Cardiovascular Risk Factor 102
   Screening for Cardiovascular Disease 102
   Importance of Modifying Vascular Risk Factors 102
   Treatment of Cardiovascular Disease 107

Diabetic Retinopathy 108
   Stages of Diabetic Retinopathy 109
   Prevention of Retinopathy 110
   Treatment of Retinopathy 111

Diabetic Renal Disease 112
   Clinical Presentation of Nephropathy 112
   Conditions that Influence Renal Function 113
   Prevention and Treatment of Diabetic Renal Disease 113

Diabetic Foot Problems 114
   Causes of Foot Problems 114
   Prevention of Foot Problems 115
   Treatment of Foot Problems 117

Neuropathic Conditions 118
   Polyneuropathy 118
   Autonomic Neuropathy 118

Other Varieties of Diabetic Neuropathy   120
Diagnosis and Treatment of Neuropathy   120

Behavior Change Strategies 123

Highlights   124

Influences on Behavior Change   125

Strategies for Behavior Change   126

Self-Management Support   127

Redesigning Practice to Support Behavior Change   128

Conclusion   129

Index 131

A Word About This Guide

Type 2 diabetes is now a worldwide epidemic. The increasing prevalence of obesity and sedentary lifestyles are driving forces in the dramatic increase of type 2 diabetes in our society. If these trends continue, one in three American children born in 2000 faces the probability of developing type 2 diabetes along with the attendant risk of morbidity and early mortality. The care of individuals with diabetes will take an increasing portion of expenditures for health care, making this disease a devastating problem for society as well as the individual. Reversing these trends will take a concerted effort in public education directed toward developing better lifestyle habits, including reduction of caloric intake and increasing exercise. The results of the Diabetes Prevention Program (DPP) and other studies have already shown that relatively small lifestyle changes can alter the transition from impaired glucose tolerance to type 2 diabetes.

Although prevention of type 2 diabetes is a necessary key to addressing the epidemic, for the foreseeable future the practitioner will be caring for an increasing number of patients with diabetes. Since the last edition of this guide, there has been a tremendous increase in our knowledge of the pathogenesis of type 2 diabetes, its complications, and the options for treatment. Numerous studies have shown that lifestyle changes and pharmacological interventions make a significant impact on the well-being of the patient. The United Kingdom Prospective Diabetes Study and several cardiovascular intervention trials have demonstrated the importance, or even preeminence, of aggressive intervention with medications to control blood pressure and lipids in addition to glucose to prevent myocardial infarction, heart failure, and peripheral arterial disease in type 2 diabetes. It is also becoming clear that when diabetes needs to be treated with medications, multiple drugs can and should be used in combination to control hyperglycemia. The addition of safe insulin sensitizers, newer insulin secretagogues, and reformulated metformin has made treatment of type 2 diabetes with oral agents easier and more effective. We have also been provided with new insulin analogs and improved delivery devices that make insulin therapy safer and easier to use. Both advances have resulted in much more widespread use of combination therapy to achieve levels of glycemic control frankly unattainable a few years ago. Using all available tools to effect behavioral change and to aggressively treat the spectrum of metabolic abnormalities associated with type 2 diabetes will likely save lives and, in the long run, decrease the cost of this disease by reducing microvascular and macrovascular complications, which contribute the bulk of the cost of caring for individuals with type 2 diabetes.

This edition of *Medical Management of Type 2 Diabetes* has been updated to provide state-of-the-art information on these issues by a select group of experts. It also reflects the most recent Clinical Practice Recommendations from the American Diabetes Association, including the new diagnostic and classification criteria adopted by the Association in 2004. This book, along with other American Diabetes Association publications, including *Medical Management of Type 1 Diabetes, Therapy for Diabetes Mellitus and Related Disorders, Intensive Diabetes Management, Medical Management of Pregnancy Complicated by Diabetes*, and *The Handbook of Diabetes and Exercise*, were designed to provide health care professionals with the comprehensive information needed to give the best possible medical care to patients with diabetes mellitus.

The American Diabetes Association believes that you will find this book as useful as its predecessors. Hopefully, it will encourage you to add other American Diabetes Association publications to your library, which can help you manage your patients with diabetes more effectively.

CHARLES F. BURANT, MD, PhD
Editor

Contributors to the Fifth Edition

EDITOR

Charles F. Burant, MD, PhD
University of Michigan
University of Michigan Diabetes
    Research and Training Center
Ann Arbor, Michigan

CONTRIBUTORS

Robert M. Anderson, EdD
University of Michigan Medical
    School
Ann Arbor, Michigan

Komel Benjamin, MPH, RD, LDN
University of North Carolina School
    of Medicine
Chapel Hill, North Carolina

John B. Buse, MD, PhD
University of North Carolina School
    of Medicine
Chapel Hill, North Carolina

Martha M. Funnell, MS, RN, CDE
University of Michigan Diabetes
    Research and Training Center
Ann Arbor, Michigan

Robin B. Nwankwo, MPH, RD,
    CDE
University of Michigan Diabetes
    Research and Training Center
Ann Arbor, Michigan

Robert E. Ratner, MD
MedStar Research Institute
Bethesda, Maryland

Martin Stevens, MD
University of Michigan Medical
    School
University of Michigan Diabetes
    Research and Training Center
Ann Arbor, Michigan

Acknowledgments

The American Diabetes Association gratefully acknowledges the contributions of the following health care professionals and members of the Association's Professional Section to previous editions of this work: Christine A. Beebe, MS, RD, CDE; Mayer B. Davidson, MD; Harold E. Lebovitz, MD; David Nathan, MD; Philip Raskin, MD; Matthew C. Riddle, MD; Harold Rifkin, MD; Robert A. Rizza, MD; F. John Service, MD, PhD; Robert Sherwin, MD; and Bruce R. Zimmerman, MD.

The Association gratefully acknowledges the reviews by Matthew C. Riddle, MD, and Nathaniel G. Clark, MD, MS, RD.

Editor Charles Burant, MD, PhD, and contributor John B. Buse, MD, PhD, acknowledge the guidance, support, teaching, and love shown by "their" mom and dad, Maria G. and John F. Buse.

Diagnosis and Classification

Highlights

Types of Diabetes Mellitus and Other Categories
  of Glucose Intolerance
   Type 1 Diabetes
   Type 2 Diabetes
   The Metabolic Syndrome
   Other Specific Types of Diabetes
   Pre-Diabetes
   Gestational Diabetes Mellitus

Screening for Diabetes Mellitus

Diagnostic Criteria for Diabetes Mellitus
   Type 1 and Type 2 Diabetes
   Pre-Diabetes
   Gestational Diabetes Mellitus

Evaluation and Classification of Patients Before Treatment

Highlights
Diagnosis and Classification

■ Diabetes mellitus has two main classifications: type 1 diabetes, which has absolute insulin deficiency and propensity to develop ketoacidosis, and type 2 diabetes, which has relative insulin deficiency combined with defects in insulin action. Type 2 diabetes is the most common form of diabetes, accounting for 90–95% of the disease in Western societies. It is most often found in overweight individuals.

■ Diabetes is diagnosed by one of the following, confirmed by repeat testing on a separate day in cases of equivocal hyperglycemia without metabolic decompensation:
- fasting plasma glucose ≥126 mg/dl (≥7.0 mmol/l)
- 2-h plasma glucose following a 75-g oral glucose tolerance test (OGTT) ≥200 mg/dl (≥11.1 mmol/l)
- random plasma glucose ≥200 mg/dl (≥11.1 mmol/l) plus symptoms of diabetes, e.g., polyuria, polydipsia, unexplained weight loss

■ Impaired fasting glucose (IFG) and impaired glucose tolerance (IGT) describe individuals with plasma glucose levels higher than normal but lower than those diagnostic for diabetes mellitus. IFG is defined as plasma glucose 100–125 mg/dl (6.1–6.9 mmol/l); IGT is plasma glucose following a 75-g OGTT 140–199 mg/dl (7.8–11.0 mmol/l).

■ Gestational diabetes mellitus (GDM), glucose intolerance first identified during pregnancy, affects ~200,000 women in the U.S. annually. As many as 50% of women with GDM later develop type 2 diabetes. Screening for GDM is recommended for women with risk factors between the 24th and 28th week of pregnancy. Diagnosis of GDM can be accomplished by either a one- or two-step approach.

■ Screening for diabetes via fasting plasma glucose should be performed every 3 years in individuals age ≥40 years. More frequent and/or earlier testing with either fasting plasma glucose or OGTT should be considered in people with additional risk factors for diabetes.

■ Beginning at age 10 years or the onset of puberty, if earlier, overweight children (≥85th percentile) should be screened every 2 years using fasting plasma glucose in the presence of any of the following: type 2 diabetes in first- or second-degree relative, high-risk ethnicity, or signs of insulin resistance, e.g., acanthosis nigricans, hypertension, dyslipidemia, polycystic ovarian syndrome.

Diagnosis and Classification

Diabetes mellitus is a chronic disorder characterized by abnormalities in the metabolism of carbohydrate, protein, and fat. Chronic, sustained exposure to these abnormalities frequently is accompanied by microvascular complications, e.g., retinopathy, neuropathy, nephropathy, as well as macrovascular complications, e.g., myocardial infarction, stroke, peripheral arterial disease. It is now recognized that diabetes mellitus encompasses a group of genetically and clinically heterogeneous disorders, in which glucose intolerance is the common denominator. Thus, although diabetes mellitus affects the metabolism of all body fuels, its diagnosis depends on identification of specific plasma glucose abnormalities.

Because the syndrome of diabetes mellitus encompasses many disorders that differ in pathogenesis, natural history, and responses to treatment, it is important that clinicians and researchers use commonly accepted terminology as well as standardized classification and diagnostic criteria when categorizing patients with glucose intolerance. In July 1997, the American Diabetes Association published diagnostic and classification criteria, replacing the criteria of the National Diabetes Data Group published in 1979. These criteria were again revised in 2003 to reflect further improvements in understanding and to correct common misunderstandings of previous recommendations.

Following the findings of the Diabetes Prevention Program, recognition of degrees of carbohydrate intolerance short of diabetes led to the description of *pre-diabetes*, a designation encompassing both states described previously as impaired fasting glucose (IFG) and impaired glucose tolerance (IGT). About 10 million people in the United States resemble the participants in the Diabetes Prevention Program in terms of age, body mass index (BMI), and glucose concentrations. If the study's interventions were implemented among such pre-diabetic people, the incidence of diabetes could be reduced substantially.

TYPES OF DIABETES MELLITUS AND OTHER CATEGORIES OF GLUCOSE INTOLERANCE

The classification of diabetes mellitus (Table 1.1) includes five clinical classes; type 1 diabetes, type 2 diabetes, other specific types of diabetes, gestational diabetes mellitus (GDM), and pre-diabetes. Hyperglycemia not sufficient to meet diagnostic criteria for diabetes was formerly characterized as IFG and IGT but is now termed *pre-diabetes* as a result of epidemiologic evidence demonstrating

Table 1.1 Types of Diabetes Mellitus and Other Categories of Abnormal Glucose Metabolism

Clinical Classification	Clinical Characteristics
Type 1 (immune-mediated) diabetes mellitus	Usually these patients have abrupt onset of polyuria and polydipsia before age 30 and present with ketosis or ketoacidosis. Although onset may be accompanied by a "honeymoon" period, they otherwise depend on insulin treatment for survival. In adulthood, the immune destruction of the pancreatic β-cells may not be severe enough to make insulin treatment essential for survival in the early stages of the disease. Patients with latent autoimmune diabetes of aging, a slow, progressive form of hyperglycemia with β-cell deterioration on an auto-immune basis, may remain independent of insulin for many years.
Type 2 diabetes mellitus	Usually these patients are age >30 yr at diagnosis, are obese or have a high percentage of abdominal fat, and have a family history of type 2 diabetes. However, along with the increase in obesity, type 2 diabetes in children and adolescents has become more common, particularly in minority populations. Because hyperglycemia at early stages may not be severe enough to cause symptoms of diabetes, many are identified during routine screening; however, complications of diabetes may be present at diagnosis. They are not prone to ketoacidosis except with severe physical stress, although children and adoles-cents may present with ketoacidosis without evidence of autoimmune destruction. The disease progresses slowly, and the treatment necessary to control hyperglycemia varies over time, including weight loss and lifestyle mod-ification, oral diabetes medications, and insulin therapy.
Gestational diabetes mellitus	These patients have glucose intolerance with onset or first recognition during pregnancy. Primary treatment is glycemic control to prevent fetal macrosomia.
Other specific types	The presentation in these patients varies, depending on the underlying disorder (Table 1.2). A careful medication and family history will help identify these patients.
Pre-diabetes	These individuals have either fasting glucose or glucose tolerance test results above normal but not diagnostic of diabetes (impaired fasting glucose or impaired glucose tolerance). Monitoring is needed for these patients, who are at increased risk of type 2 diabetes and cardiovascu-lar disease. Lifestyle modification or therapy with met-formin or acarbose has been found to prevent or delay progression to diabetes.

an association of macrovascular complications with these less extreme levels of carbohydrate intolerance, together with the frequent progression to diabetes.

The current classification recognizes that a specific type of diabetes may have different stages with varying degrees of hyperglycemia and that classification should not be determined by the degree or treatment of hyperglycemia. Two observations have made classification of diabetes more problematic. First, recognition of latent autoimmune diabetes of aging (LADA), accounting for as much as 10–15% of new onset diabetes among adults, alters our perception of pathogenesis of diabetes occurring in this age-group. LADA presents as a slow, progressive form of hyperglycemia with β-cell deterioration on an autoimmune basis. Individuals with LADA may remain insulin independent for many years but share pathogenic features with people who have traditional autoimmune type 1 diabetes. Second, the epidemic of type 2 diabetes in children and adolescents has altered the demographics of diabetes in these age-groups. Type 2 diabetes now accounts for 25–33% of all cases of diabetes in children and adolescents, particularly in ethnic minority populations. Although these individuals may present with diabetic ketoacidosis, no evidence exists of active autoimmunity or β-cell destruction. Many of these individuals subsequently are able to stop insulin therapy and control hyperglycemia with lifestyle modifications with or without oral antidiabetic agents.

TYPE 1 DIABETES

Type 1 diabetes previously was called insulin-dependent diabetes mellitus (IDDM), type I diabetes, or juvenile-onset diabetes. There are two subgroups of type 1 diabetes: the more common immune-mediated class and an unusual idiopathic class. Patients with type 1 diabetes have severe insulinopenia and are prone to ketoacidosis. At diagnosis, type 1 patients usually are lean, have experienced recent weight loss and symptoms of excessive thirst and urination, and are ketonuric or in ketoacidosis. In the stage of complete evolution of the disease, patients with type 1 diabetes depend on exogenous insulin to prevent ketoacidosis and death.

Type 1 diabetes is estimated to account for 5–10% of all known cases of diabetes mellitus in the U.S. The exact prevalence remains to be established but is almost certainly <0.5% of the population; it is lower among nonwhite than white populations. Although type 1 diabetes may occur at any age, the peak of onset occurs at the time of puberty. Many Hispanic/Latino, African-American, and Native American youths with onset of diabetes before age 20 have type 2 diabetes.

Type 1 immune-mediated diabetes mellitus has strong human leukocyte antigen (HLA) associations, indicating an inherited predisposition to the disease. Early in the disease process, markers of immune destruction of the β-cell are found, including islet cell autoantibodies (ICAs), autoantibodies to insulin (IAAs), and autoantibodies to glutamic acid decarboxylase (GAD). β-Cell destruction occurs at varying rates, usually more rapidly in younger patients, which accounts for the usual abrupt, classic clinical manifestations, and more slowly in adults, which may lead to the mistaken clinical classification of type 2 diabetes. Patients with LADA, a slow, progressive form of hyperglycemia with β-cell deterioration on an autoimmune basis, may remain independent of insulin for many years. In adults, anti-GAD is the most frequently positive immune marker and is positive in approximately two of three cases and thus may be useful in diagnosing LADA in patients whose classification is in doubt.

TYPE 2 DIABETES

Type 2 diabetes, previously referred to as non-insulin-dependent diabetes mellitus (NIDDM), type II diabetes, or adult-onset diabetes, is a progressive disorder characterized by variable degrees of insulin resistance and progressive β-cell dysfunction, leading to a relative and, in some individuals, an absolute deficiency of insulin secretion. As many as one-third to one-half of these individuals ultimately require insulin therapy to control hyperglycemia. Thus, the old classifications of diabetes that were based on insulin dependency frequently confused this large subset with people who had type 1 diabetes. Current classification is intended to avoid this confusion.

Type 2 diabetes disproportionately affects Native Americans, African Americans, Hispanics/Latinos, and Asian American/Pacific Islanders, and the increased prevalence in these ethnic groups appears to be associated with a westernized diet and concomitant obesity. Type 2 diabetes affects ~17 million Americans, over 6% of the population. The incidence of type 2 diabetes is growing in epidemic proportions not only in the United States, but worldwide, likely as the result of changes in human behavior and lifestyle during the last 100 years. In particular, the increase in diabetes seems to be caused by sedentary lifestyles and obesity. According to World Health Organization estimates, >300 million individuals may have diabetes by the year 2025.

Type 2 diabetes in children and adolescents has become an epidemic, particularly in minority populations. Although these children may present with ketoacidosis, no evidence is seen of active autoimmunity or β-cell destruction. Many children and adolescents can discontinue insulin therapy and be maintained with lifestyle modifications, with or without oral antidiabetic agents.

The following are characteristics of type 2 diabetes:

- Type 2 diabetes is associated with defects in both insulin secretion and insulin action.
- Type 2 diabetes can occur at any age, but usually is diagnosed after age 30.
- The age of clinical presentation may be decreasing in some ethnic groups.
- Although ~80% of patients are obese or have a history of obesity at the time of diagnosis, type 2 diabetes can occur in nonobese individuals, especially in the elderly.
- Patients with type 2 diabetes may or may not present with the classic symptoms of diabetes mellitus, e.g., polydipsia, polyuria, polyphagia, weight loss.
- Patients with type 2 diabetes are not prone to develop ketoacidosis except during periods of severe stress, such as those caused by infections, trauma, medications, or surgery.
- Patients with type 2 diabetes frequently present with microvascular and macrovascular chronic complications of diabetes.

The precise etiology of type 2 diabetes remains unknown. It appears to be a heterogeneous disorder, with genetics and environment playing a role in most individuals. Identical twin studies indicate that there is >75% concordance for this disease, but the exact genes that predispose an individual to diabetes have not been defined. Unlike type 1 diabetes, circulating islet cell antibodies are not present.

Intake of excessive calories, leading to weight gain and obesity, probably is an important factor in the pathogenesis of type 2 diabetes. In fact, obesity, particularly visceral obesity, has been singled out as a powerful risk factor in type 2 diabetes, and even small weight losses are associated with a change in plasma glucose levels toward normal in many patients. A sedentary lifestyle also has been linked to an increased propensity to develop type 2 diabetes. The insulin resistance syndrome, hyperinsulinemia, and IGT are also all strong risk factors for developing type 2 diabetes, as is previous GDM. The Diabetes Prevention Program and similar studies have demonstrated the ability to identify high-risk individuals and delay or prevent the progression to type 2 diabetes.

THE METABOLIC SYNDROME

Type 2 diabetes and pre-diabetes are, in most instances, manifestations of a significant underlying disorder known as the metabolic syndrome. Originally described by Reaven to include insulin resistance, glucose intolerance, hyperinsulinemia, increased triglyceride and decreased HDL cholesterol levels, and hypertension, additional abnormalities are now considered part of the syndrome, including increased body weight (especially central adiposity), inflammation, microalbuminuria, hyperuricemia, abnormalities of fibrinolysis and coagulation, polycystic ovary syndrome, and nonalcoholic fatty liver disease. It has been suggested that insulin resistance underlies the pathogenesis of many or all of these metabolic abnormalities. Individuals with the metabolic syndrome are at significant risk of developing type 2 diabetes and cardiovascular disease. No uniform definition of the metabolic syndrome exists, but there are similarities between that proposed by the World Health Organization, which includes the presence of insulin resistance, and that of the National Cholesterol Education Program Adult Treatment Panel III (ATP III), which does not include a measure of insulin resistance (Table 1.2). Data from the third National Health and Nutrition Examination Survey, which used the ATP III criteria, found that the overall prevalence of the metabolic syndrome in the U.S. a decade ago was ~25%. The incidence in different ethnic populations varies depending on the criteria but is highest in Mexican Americans. The prevalence rises with age at least into the seventh decade, reaching ~50%.

OTHER SPECIFIC TYPES OF DIABETES

This category contains the smallest number of patients and may represent <3% of people with diabetes. Table 1.3 lists the disorders included in this category. Although this is a small subset of patients with diabetes, correct identification of these patients is important because the treatment often differs. Recognition of patients in this group requires clinical alertness to identify the examination features or historical differences that lead to the correct diagnosis.

In the previous classification system, there were families in which diabetes was present in children, adolescents, and adults and in which an autosomal-dominant inheritance had been established. This form of diabetes was referred to as maturity-onset diabetes of the young (MODY) and was considered a subtype of type 2 diabetes. In the new classification system, MODY resides in the group "other specific

Table 1.2 Criteria for Diagnosis of the Metabolic Syndrome

World Health Organization Criteria

Presence of diabetes, impaired glucose tolerance, impaired fasting glucose, or insulin resistance plus two or more of the following abnormalities:

- High blood pressure: ≥160/90 mmHg
- Dyslipidemia: triglyceride concentration ≥150 mg/dl (≥1.695 mmol/l) and/or HDL cholesterol <35 mg/dl (<0.9 mmol/l) in men and <39 mg/dl (<1.0 mmol/l) in women
- Central obesity: waist-to-hip ratio >0.90 in men or >0.85 in women and/or BMI >30 kg/m²
- Microalbuminuria: urinary albumin excretion rate ≥20 µg/min or albumin-to-creatinine ratio ≥20 mg/g

ATP III Criteria

Presence of three or more of the following abnormalities:

- High blood pressure: ≥130/85 mmHg
- Hypertriglyceridemia: ≥150 mg/dl (≥1.695 mmol/l)
- Low HDL cholesterol: <40 mg/dl (<1.036 mmol/l) in men and <50 mg/dl (<1.295 mmol/l) in women
- Abdominal obesity: waist circumference >102 cm in men and >88 cm in women
- High fasting glucose: ≥110 mg/dl (≥6.1 mmol/l)

Adapted from Ford and Giles. ATP III, National Cholesterol Education Program Expert Panel on Detection, Evaluation, and Treatment of High Blood Cholesterol in Adults (Adult Treatment Panel III).

types," because there are distinct genetic defects of β-cell function responsible for these types of diabetes and there are minimal or no defects in insulin action, the hallmark of type 2 diabetes. To date, abnormalities of six different functional genes on different chromosomes have been identified that cause MODY. Each abnormality leads to impaired insulin secretion. Numerous other specific mutations have also been identified in insulin, the insulin receptor, and mitochondrial DNA, which result in the development of diabetes.

The new classification has also removed "malnutrition-related diabetes," because no evidence exists that protein deficiency causes diabetes. Many patients previously in this class have fibrocalculous pancreatopathy as the cause of their diabetes. This form of diabetes is common in tropical countries but is rare in the United States.

PRE-DIABETES

IFG (fasting plasma glucose [FPG] 100–125 mg/dl [6.1–6.9 mmol/l]) and IGT (2-h sample after 75-g oral glucose tolerance test [OGTT] 140–199 mg/dl [7.8–11.0 mmol/l]) describe individuals who have plasma glucose levels that are higher than normal but lower than those diagnostic for diabetes mellitus. The importance of this category is that it represents a risk factor for future diabetes and cardiovascular disease. These patients do not develop the microvascular complications of diabetes unless their hyperglycemia progresses to levels diagnostic

Table 1.3 Other Specific Types of Diabetes Mellitus

- Genetic defects of β-cell function
  - Chromosome 20, hepatic nuclear factor (HNF)-4α (MODY1)
  - Chromosome 7, glucokinase (MODY2)
  - Chromosome 12, HNF-1α (MODY3)
  - Insulin promoter factor-1 (MODY4)
  - HNF-1 β (MODY5)
  - NeuroD1/BETA2 (MODY6)
  - Mitochondrial DNA
  - Mutant insulins
  - Hyperproinsulinemia
  - Others
- Genetic defects in insulin action
  - Type A insulin resistance
  - Leprechaunism
  - Rabson-Mendenhall syndrome
  - Lipoatrophic diabetes
  - Others
- Diseases of the exocrine pancreas
  - Pancreatitis
  - Trauma/pancreatectomy
  - Neoplasia
  - Cystic fibrosis
  - Hemochromatosis
  - Fibrocalculous pancreatopathy
  - Others
- Endocrinopathies
  - Acromegaly
  - Cushing's syndrome
  - Glucagonoma
  - Pheochromocytoma
  - Hyperthyroidism
  - Somatostatinoma
  - Aldosteronoma
  - Others
- Drug- or chemical-induced
  - Vacor
  - Pentamidine
  - Nicotinic acid
  - Glucocorticoids
  - Thyroid hormone
  - Diazoxide
  - β-Adrenergic agonists
  - Thiazides
  - Dilantin
  - α-Interferon
  - Protease inhibitors (e.g., indinavir, saquinavir, ritonavir, nelfinavir)
  - Atypical antipsychotics (e.g., clozapine, olanzapine, quetiapine, risperidone)
  - Others
- Infections
  - Congenital rubella
  - Cytomegalovirus
  - Others
- Uncommon forms of immune-mediated diabetes
  - "Stiff-man" syndrome
  - Anti-insulin receptor antibodies
  - Others
- Other genetic syndromes sometimes associated with diabetes
  - Down's syndrome
  - Klinefelter's syndrome
  - Wolfram's syndrome
  - Friedreich's ataxia
  - Huntington's chorea
  - Laurence-Moon-Biedl syndrome
  - Myotonic dystrophy
  - Porphyria
  - Prader-Willi syndrome
  - Others

of diabetes. The Diabetes Prevention Program and other studies demonstrated that lifestyle modifications—dietary modification to reduce weight by 5–10% and moderately vigorous physical activity for at least 30 min most days of the week—prevents or delays the onset of diabetes in people with pre-diabetes. The use of drug therapy to prevent the development of diabetes is controversial. Two studies have examined the use of metformin to prevent the development of diabetes, with mixed results: metformin seems to prevent or delay the onset of diabetes in those who are very overweight (BMI >34 kg/m^2) and in younger subjects, particularly those under age 40. Two studies have examined the effect of acarbose on the development of diabetes, with consistent results: acarbose seems to moderately reduce the risk of developing diabetes. Orlistat, a weight loss product, has been evaluated in one study and demonstrated to reduce the risk of developing diabetes in people with IGT. Two studies have demonstrated a substantial effect of troglitazone to prevent or delay diabetes. Although it is likely that the available thiazolidinediones, pioglitazone and rosiglitazone, provide some protection from diabetes due to their insulin-sensitizing effects, the extent of this protection will only be clarified by ongoing clinical studies.

The American Diabetes Association recommends lifestyle intervention in patients with pre-diabetes. There are insufficient data to routinely recommend drug therapy to prevent diabetes, because the long-term benefits and risks of these approaches are not yet adequately known. Clearly, careful assessment and aggressive treatment of cardiovascular risk factors are appropriate due to the increased risk of cardiovascular disease in this population.

GESTATIONAL DIABETES MELLITUS

The term *gestational diabetes mellitus* is used to describe glucose intolerance that is first detected during pregnancy. Women with known diabetes mellitus before conception are not part of this class. GDM affects ~4–7% of pregnancies, about 200,000 American women, annually, usually during the second or third trimester, when levels of insulin-antagonist hormones increase and insulin resistance occurs. Normally, increased insulin secretion compensates for the insulin resistance. Up to 50% of women with GDM later develop type 2 diabetes, about 5–10% of whom are diagnosed in the postpartum period.

SCREENING FOR DIABETES MELLITUS

The prevalence of undiagnosed diabetes mellitus in the United States is ~3% of the population, and the currently recommended diagnostic tests for diabetes are neither 100% specific nor 100% sensitive. Based on these facts, it is generally agreed that the risk to the patient of inappropriate diagnosis outweighs the benefits to be gained from screening tests for diabetes in the general community. However, screening high-risk individuals is appropriate. High-risk individuals can be identified through data on various demographic, physical, historical, and laboratory parameters.

The recommended screening test for nonpregnant adults is an FPG determination. Evaluation for diabetes mellitus should be limited to nonpregnant individuals with a high risk of developing diabetes, and guidelines exist for identifying those who should be screened and when (Table 1.4).

Screening pregnant women for GDM is important because 60,000–90,000 women with the disease give birth each year and GDM is associated with increased perinatal morbidity. Screening for GDM normally is done between the 24th and 28th week of pregnancy. The small subset of women who are age <25 years, are of normal body weight, have no first-degree relatives with diabetes, and are Caucasian have a low risk of GDM and need not be screened. This exclusion from screening represents a change from the previous recommendation to screen all pregnant women.

Table 1.4 Candidates for Diabetes Screening

- Testing for diabetes should be considered in all individuals at age ≥45 years, particularly in those with BMI ≥25 kg/m²* and, if normal, should be repeated at 3-year intervals.
- Testing should be considered at a younger age or be carried out more frequently in individuals who are overweight (BMI ≥25 kg/m²*) and have additional risk factors:
  - Are habitually physically inactive
  - Have a first-degree relative with diabetes
  - Are members of a high-risk ethnic population, e.g., African American, Latino, Native American, Asian American, Pacific Islander
  - Have delivered a baby weighing >9 lb or have been diagnosed with GDM
  - Are hypertensive (>140/90 mmHg)
  - Have HDL cholesterol level ≤35 mg/dl (≤0.90 mmol/l) and/or triglyceride level >250 mg/dl (>2.82 mmol/l)
  - Have polycystic ovary syndrome (PCOS)
  - On previous testing, had IGT or IFG
  - Have other clinical conditions associated with insulin resistance, e.g., PCOS, acanthosis nigricans
  - Have a history of vascular disease

*May not be correct for all ethnic groups.

After parturition, patients with GDM should be followed closely. In most cases, glucose tolerance in women with GDM returns to normal after delivery. Within 5–15 years after parturition, however, 40–60% of women with GDM develop type 2 diabetes.

DIAGNOSTIC CRITERIA FOR DIABETES MELLITUS

TYPE 1 AND TYPE 2 DIABETES

A diagnosis of diabetes can be made on the basis of a random plasma glucose concentration plus signs and symptoms of diabetes, an FPG concentration, or a properly performed OGTT. Diagnostic criteria for diabetes are presented in Table 1.5.

The FPG is the test of choice because of its simplicity, accuracy, and reproducibility. The diagnostic level for diabetes is ≥126 mg/dl (≥7.0 mmol/l). The diagnostic levels selected also have been shown in several studies to be very close to the cutoff points at which microvascular complications of diabetes begin to develop, providing some validity for the importance of this degree of hyperglycemia. Although positive urine glucose tests are strongly suggestive of diabetes in symptomatic patients, they should never be used for the definitive diagnosis of diabetes mellitus.

The OGTT is useful only if performed with strict adherence to proper methods, including assurance of a diet adequate in carbohydrate, i.e., 150 g/day for 3 days; absence of underlying illness; and absence of interfering drugs.

Table 1.5 Diagnostic Criteria for Diabetes Mellitus

- Symptoms of diabetes plus casual plasma glucose concentration ≥200 mg/dl (≥11.1 mmol/l). Casual is defined as any time of day without regard to time since last meal. The classic symptoms of diabetes include polyuria, polydipsia, and unexplained weight loss.

  or
- FPG ≥126 mg/dl (≥7.0 mmol/l). Fasting is defined as no caloric intake for at least 8 h.

  or
- 2-h plasma glucose ≥200 mg/dl (≥11.1 mmol/l) during an OGTT. The test should be performed as described by the World Health Organization using a glucose load containing the equivalent of 75 g anhydrous glucose dissolved in water administered in the fasting state after 3 days of adequate carbohydrate intake.

In the absence of unequivocal hyperglycemia with acute metabolic decompensation, these criteria should be confirmed by repeat testing on a different day.

OGTTs have been used extensively to establish the incidence and prevalence of diabetes in population-based studies. However, OGTTs are of limited value in making the diagnosis of diabetes in a given individual because of the variability from test to test. The OGTT should not be performed if FPG is ≥126 mg/dl (≥7.0 mmol/l).

The OGTT is performed using a 75-g oral glucose load. Intermediate time point determinations are no longer used for diagnosis during the OGTT; rather, the 2-h plasma glucose value alone is used.

PRE-DIABETES

Some patients do not meet these criteria, but their test results are not completely normal either. They are classified as having pre-diabetes:

- IFG = FPG ≥100 to <126 mg/dl (≥5.6 to <7.0 mmol/l)
- IGT = 2-h OGTT plasma glucose ≥140 to <200 mg/dl (≥7.8 to <11.1 mmol/l)

GESTATIONAL DIABETES MELLITUS

A screening test is recommended using a 50-g oral glucose load, followed by a 1-h plasma glucose measurement, for most pregnant women. The patient need not be fasting for this test. A value ≥130 mg/dl (≥7.2 mmol/l) has 90% sensitivity for detecting GDM, and a value ≥140 mg/dl (≥7.8 mmol/l) has 80% sensitivity for detecting GDM by the "gold standard": 3-h 100-g OGTT. Because of the uncertainty, some do not perform the screening test and proceed directly to the diagnostic procedure. Table 1.5 lists the diagnostic criteria for the 3-h 100-g OGTT and the alternative 2-h 75-g OGTT. During normal pregnancy, FPG levels tend to decrease, whereas postglucose load levels tend to increase. Thus, criteria for diag-

Table 1.6 Diagnosis of Gestational Diabetes Mellitus

After a 100-g oral glucose load, diagnosis of GDM may be made if two plasma glucose values equal or exceed:

Fasting	95 mg/dl (5.3 mmol/l)
1-h	180 mg/dl (10.0 mmol/l)
2-h	155 mg/dl (8.6 mmol/l)
3-h	140 mg/dl (7.8 mmol/l)

After a 75-g oral glucose load, diagnosis of GDM may be made if two plasma glucose values equal or exceed:

Fasting	95 mg/dl (5.3 mmol/l)
1-h	180 mg/dl (10.0 mmol/l)
2-h	155 mg/dl (8.6 mmol/l)

nosis of GDM are adjusted appropriately and are calculated to provide maximum sensitivity to diagnose diabetes during pregnancy. Exceeding two or more of the glucose concentrations noted in Table 1.6 has been demonstrated to increase risk to the fetus.

EVALUATION AND CLASSIFICATION OF PATIENTS BEFORE TREATMENT

Before therapy is initiated to treat diabetes mellitus, the patient should have a complete medical evaluation and be classified appropriately. The complete medical evaluation helps the physician classify the patient, determine the possible presence of underlying diseases that may require further study, detect the presence of complications frequently associated with diabetes mellitus (see Chapter 5, Detection and Treatment of Chronic Complications), assist in formulating a management plan, and provide a basis for continuing care. See Table 1.7 for a complete list for an initial medical evaluation, regardless of when diabetes was diagnosed.

The patient should not be classified until all data necessary for making the determination are available. Generally, a reasonably good initial assignment of the patient can be made on the basis of a complete personal and family history and diagnostic test results. The most important distinguishing characteristics of diabetes mellitus are presented in Table 1.1. Patients should not be classified on the basis of age alone or on whether or not they are taking insulin therapy. If the diagnosis of diabetes had been made previously, an initial evaluation should also review the previous treatment and the past and present degrees of glycemic control. Laboratory tests appropriate to the evaluation of each patient's general medical condition should be performed.

A major problem in classification is that it is sometimes difficult to assign the patient to a particular type of diabetes mellitus (i.e., type 1 or type 2). For example,

Table 1.7 Complete Initial Evaluation for Diabetes

Medical History

- Symptoms
- Results of laboratory tests and special examination results related to the diagnosis of diabetes
- Prior A1C records
- Eating patterns, nutritional status, and weight history; growth and development in children and adolescents
- Details of previous treatment programs, including nutrition and diabetes self-management education, attitudes, and health beliefs
- Current treatment of diabetes, including medications, meal plan, and results of glucose monitoring and patient's use of data
- Exercise history
- Frequency, severity, and cause of acute complications, such as ketoacidosis and hypoglycemia
- Prior or current infections, particularly skin, foot, dental, and genitourinary
- Symptoms and treatment of chronic complications associated with diabetes, including eye, kidney, nerve, genito-urinary (including sexual), bladder, gastrointestinal (including symptoms of celiac disease in type 1 diabetes patients), heart, peripheral arterial, and cerebrovascular function and feet
- Other medications that may affect blood glucose levels
- Risk factors for atherosclerosis: smoking, hypertension, obesity, dyslipidemia, and family history
- History and treatment of other conditions, including endocrine and eating disorders
- Family history of diabetes and other endocrine disorders
- Lifestyle, cultural, psychosocial, educational, and economic factors that may influence the management of diabetes
- Tobacco, alcohol, and/or controlled substance use
- Contraception and reproductive and sexual history

Physical Examination

- Height and weight (and comparison to norms in children and adolescents)
- Sexual maturation (during peripubertal period)
- Blood pressure determination, including orthostatic measurements when indicated, and comparison to age-related norms
- Fundoscopic examination
- Oral examination
- Thyroid palpation
- Cardiac examination
- Abdominal examination, e.g., for hepatomegaly
- Evaluation of pulses by palpitation and with auscultation
- Hand/finger examination
- Foot examination
- Skin examination for acanthosis nigricans and insulin injection sites
- Neurological examination
- Signs of diseases that can cause secondary diabetes, e.g., hemochromatosis, pancreatic disease

Laboratory Evaluation

- A1C
- Fasting lipid profile, including total cholesterol, HDL cholesterol, triglycerides, and LDL cholesterol
- Test for microalbuminuria in type 1 diabetes patients who have had diabetes for at least 5 years and in all patients with type 2 diabetes. Some advocate beginning screening of pubertal children before 5 years of diabetes.
- Serum creatinine in adults and in children if proteinuria is present
- Thyroid-stimulating hormone (TSH) in all type 1 diabetes patients and in type 2 diabetes patients if clinically indicated
- Electrocardiogram in adults

(continued)

Table 1.7 Complete Initial Evaluation for Diabetes (*continued*)

- Urinalysis for ketones, protein, and sediment
- Microalbumin-to-urine creatinine ratio

Referrals

- Eye examination, if indicated
- Family planning for women of reproductive potential

- Medical nutrition therapy, as indicated
- Diabetes educator, if not provided by physician or practice staff
- Behavioral specialist, as indicated
- Foot specialist, as indicated
- Other specialties and services as appropriate

A1C, glycated hemoglobin A$_{1c}$.

the normal-weight type 2 patient who has been taking insulin often appears to be a type 1 patient. Another example is the newly diagnosed child or adolescent who is a member of a family with an autosomal-dominant form of inheritance of diabetes, such as in MODY, where there is a genetic defect of the β-cell. Such a patient should not be classified as having type 1 diabetes on the basis of age alone. Some patients with characteristics of type 2 diabetes require insulin therapy for glycemic control but do not depend on insulin to prevent ketoacidosis or to sustain life. These patients should not be classified as having type 1 diabetes simply on the basis of their insulin regimen. Other patients, particularly adults, have type 1 immune-mediated diabetes but are at a stage in which they still have β-cell function and clinically appear similar to those with typical type 2 diabetes. It usually is not necessary for clinicians to determine the presence of islet cell or other antibodies or the degree of insulin secretion, but if this problem is suspected, these measurements may be helpful. There is some evidence that these patients do better when treated with insulin, even though they may temporarily respond to an oral agent. The measurement of stimulated plasma C-peptide levels after oral or intravenous stimulus often is used as an index of insulin secretion; however, it has not proved to be a useful classification tool for routine use, particularly at diagnosis. After 5 years of insulin therapy, most patients with autoimmune type 1 diabetes will have C-peptide levels at or near the lower limits of normal for the assay. A history of diabetic ketoacidosis is no longer a highly specific marker of type 1 diabetes. Perhaps the most specific markers of type 1 diabetes at presentation are weight loss and ketonuria and, during treatment with insulin, highly erratic glycemic control. Although the classification of some patients may thus be problematic, the goal of therapy remains the achievement of near-normal glycemia.

BIBLIOGRAPHY

American Diabetes Association: Diagnosis and classification of diabetes mellitus. *Diabetes Care* 27 (Suppl. 1):S5–S10, 2004

Ananth J, Venkatesh R, Burgoyne K, Gunatilake S: Atypical antipsychotic drug use and diabetes. *Psychother Psychosom* 71:244–254, 2002

Diabetes Prevention Program Research Group: Reduction in the incidence of type 2 diabetes with lifestyle intervention or metformin. *N Engl J Med* 346:393–403, 2002

Florez JC, Hirschhorn J, Altshuler D: The inherited basis of diabetes mellitus: implications for the genetic analysis of complex traits (Review). *Annu Rev Genomics Hum Genet* 4:257–291, 2003

Ford ES, Giles WH: A comparison of the prevalence of the metabolic syndrome using two proposed definitions. *Diabetes Care* 26:575–581, 2003

Stern MP, Williams K, Haffner SM: Identification of persons at high risk for type 2 diabetes mellitus: do we need the oral glucose tolerance test? *Ann Intern Med* 136:575–581, 2002

World Health Organization: *Diabetes Mellitus: Report of a WHO Study Group.* Geneva, World Health Org., 1985 (Tech. Rep. Ser., no. 727)

Zimmet P, Alberti KG, Shaw J: Global and societal implications of the diabetes epidemic. *Nature* 414:782–787, 2001

Pathogenesis

Highlights

Genetic and Environmental Factors

Insulin Resistance
Sites of Insulin Resistance
Mechanisms of Insulin Resistance

The Fat Cell as an Endocrine Organ

Defects in Insulin Secretion
Factors Modulating Insulin Secretion
Physiological Consequences of Defective Insulin Secretion

Conclusion

Highlights
Pathogenesis

■ Type 2 diabetes develops because of excessive caloric intake for a given level of activity in a genetically predisposed individual.

■ The genetic cause of diabetes has been identified in only a small fraction of individuals with type 2 diabetes. Likely, the genetic risk is produced by the interaction of multiple genes, each of which confers a risk for the development of the disease.

■ Defects in insulin action and insulin secretion are seen in most individuals with type 2 diabetes.

■ Skeletal muscle, liver, and adipose tissue are the primary sites of insulin resistance.

■ β-Cell dysfunction leading to a relative decrease in insulin levels is a progressive process and likely results from intrinsic secretion failure and decreases in β-cell mass.

■ Abnormalities in the uptake and metabolism of fatty acid in peripheral tissues and in the β-cells may be a primary event in the development of insulin resistance and β-cell failure.

Pathogenesis

Type 2 diabetes is a chronic disorder characterized by diminished liver, muscle, and adipose tissue sensitivity to insulin, termed *insulin resistance*, and a superimposed impairment of β-cell secretory function. Although abnormal carbohydrate metabolism is the defining disorder, changes in fat and protein metabolism clearly occur and contribute to the complications arising from this progressive metabolic disease. Type 2 diabetes is the most common form of diabetes, accounting for >90% of cases. In most cases, the development of type 2 diabetes is due to environmental influences on a susceptible genetic background. Worldwide, the incidence of diabetes is rising rapidly due to modernization and the resultant access to greater quantities of foodstuffs and modern conveniences that lead to increased caloric consumption and decreased energy expenditure.

GENETIC AND ENVIRONMENTAL FACTORS

Multiple lines of evidence show that type 2 diabetes is a genetic disease. The incidence of type 2 diabetes is especially high among certain ethnic populations such as Hispanics/Latinos, Aboriginal peoples in the Americas and Australia, Pacific and Indian Ocean island populations, and the peoples of the Indian subcontinent. A family history of type 2 diabetes is another important risk factor for the development of diabetes. Specific genetic aberrations are present in only small subpopulations with type 2 diabetes, such as that seen in maturity-onset diabetes of the young (MODY).

For most, the genetic risk is due to interactions between multiple genes, each of which can protect or sensitize an individual to the consequence of increased food intake and decreased physical activity. Variations in the amino acid sequence of proteins have been linked to the susceptibility to develop diabetes, but the way in which these genetic variations interact to predispose an individual to diabetes has not been determined. Thus, with the exception of the rare forms of type 2 diabetes, a test that would predict genetic susceptibility is not available.

The genes that predispose an individual to diabetes have likely been selected through evolution. Until recently, humans have lived in a relatively nutrient-poor environment. Possessing genes that allow for the efficient accumulation and storage of nutrients would be a distinct advantage during times of chronic or intermittent food shortage. However, these so-called "thrifty genes" are maladaptive in today's consistently food-rich environment.

At present, there is no clear indication that ingestion of a certain type of nutrient, whether carbohydrate, fat, or protein, independent of total caloric intake is more harmful in respect to the development of diabetes. The combination of a sedentary lifestyle with an increased caloric intake leading to weight gain and the development of obesity is the primary factor in the development of insulin resistance and, ultimately, type 2 diabetes.

INSULIN RESISTANCE

Insulin resistance is defined as a decrease in the activity of endogenous or exogenously administered insulin to alter metabolism in target tissues. Insulin resistance is a consistent finding in patients with type 2 diabetes, and resistance is present years before the onset of diabetes and predicts the onset of diabetes. Most individuals are able to maintain normal glucose levels by increasing β-cell insulin production to compensate for the decrease in insulin action. However, in susceptible individuals, increasing insulin resistance or a failure of β-cells to maintain high levels of insulin secretion leads to progressive glucose intolerance and subsequent diabetes. It is likely that genetics plays a role both in the propensity to develop insulin resistance and in the risk for β-cell failure in response to insulin resistance.

SITES OF INSULIN RESISTANCE

Insulin resistance exists in both hepatic and peripheral tissues. Skeletal muscle is the primary site of glucose uptake after a meal and is the primary site of insulin resistance. Decreases in skeletal muscle glucose uptake and nonoxidative disposal (predominantly glycogen synthesis) are the main findings in diabetes. The decrease in insulin-mediated muscle glucose disposal contributes to the excessive rise in plasma glucose concentration after a mixed meal in patients with type 2 diabetes. Adipose tissue also shows resistance to insulin-stimulated glucose uptake as well as resistance to inhibition of lypolysis.

In the liver, insulin resistance leads to a failure to suppress hepatic glucose production, even in the face of fasting hyperinsulinemia. Basal rates of hepatic glucose production are increased when the fasting plasma glucose exceeds 110 mg/dl (6.1 mmol/l). Increases in hepatic glucose production directly correlate with the level of fasting plasma glucose. Patients with type 2 diabetes do not demonstrate normal suppression of hepatic glucose output when insulin is infused intravenously at a low concentration. At high infusion concentrations of insulin, hepatic glucose output can be suppressed, indicating a partial ability to overcome the insulin resistance.

MECHANISMS OF INSULIN RESISTANCE

The action of insulin on its target tissues is influenced by sex, age, ethnicity, physical activity, medications, and, most important, weight. Insulin resistance is known to be present to some degree in most obese individuals and is found in most individuals with type 2 diabetes. The degree of obesity, as manifested by the body mass index (BMI), correlates well with the degree of insulin resistance and with the

risk for type 2 diabetes. The relationship between BMI and diabetes risk is different among ethnic populations. For example, the risk for diabetes occurs at a lower BMI in Asian individuals than in most other ethnic groups.

The development of obesity commonly results in an accumulation of intra-abdominal fat, which may be a stronger predictor of type 2 diabetes than overall BMI. Intra-abdominal fat is metabolically distinct from subcutaneous tissue. It is more lipolytically active and less sensitive to the antilipolytic effects of insulin. This results in increases in the flux of free fatty acids (FFAs) from the fat to the liver and to the periphery. Despite increased flux, serum FFAs may not be markedly elevated due to efficient extraction by the liver and skeletal muscle. Excess delivery of FFAs stimulates liver glucose production, decreases skeletal muscle insulin sensitivity, and results in blunted insulin release as well as affecting vascular reactivity and coagulation parameters.

The cellular processes that are affected in the muscle, liver, and β-cells leading to insulin resistance are becoming clarified, but the exact mechanisms remain to be determined. In muscle, a small reduction in insulin binding to its cell surface receptor is observed in type 2 diabetes and is due to downregulation of the receptor in response to hyperinsulinemia. Although abnormal insulin binding associated with mutations in the insulin gene and the insulin receptor gene have significant insulin resistance, it is not thought that the changes associated with type 2 diabetes are of sufficient magnitude to result in the degree of insulin resistance commonly seen.

Postreceptor abnormalities are primarily responsible for insulin resistance in the skeletal muscle and liver in patients with type 2 diabetes. After binding insulin, the insulin receptor initiates a complex cascade of protein phosphorylations and dephosphorylations and other processes that result in various cellular events. Increases, decreases, and aberrant phosphorylation of specific proteins, including the insulin receptor, results in impaired propagation of signals. This decreases the translocation of the glucose transporter proteins from the cytoplasm to the cell membrane, resulting in decreased glucose transport. There are also defects in activation of glycogen synthesis as well as impaired mitochondrial oxidation of substrates.

In the liver, elevated FFAs may antagonize the effects of insulin to suppress endogenous glucose production. There is a direct relationship between fasting blood glucose and the resistance of the liver to insulin. Peripheral insulin resistance may also play a role in the increased glucose production by the liver. The inability of insulin to suppress the mobilization of gluconeogenic precursors from peripheral tissue results in their increased delivery to the liver and stimulation of gluconeogenesis.

In both muscle and liver, the accumulation of intracellular stores of triglyceride strongly correlates with the degree of insulin resistance. This is likely a marker of an inequality of fatty acid delivery (or synthesis in the liver) and the ability of these tissues to oxidize the fats. This process leads to the buildup of long-chain acyl-CoA molecules, which can act as signaling molecules. The accumulation of the acyl-CoA molecules is exacerbated by glucose and its metabolites, which can lead to decreases in fatty acid import into the mitochondria and decreasing oxidation.

Another theory for the accumulation of triglyceride stores in peripheral tissue in insulin-resistant individuals and those with type 2 diabetes is the "overflow" hypothesis. This theory suggests that the ability to expand adipose mass is limited and the excess energy "overflows" into other tissues, disrupting normal metabolism. An extreme example of this phenomenon is seen in individuals with lipodystrophy, who have a partial or complete absence of adipose tissue. These individuals develop extreme insulin resistance, elevated serum triglyceride and FFA levels, accumulation of "ectopic" triglyceride stores in muscle and liver associated with steatosis, inflammation, and cirrhosis. The same abnormalities are found in many with type 2 diabetes.

THE FAT CELL AS AN ENDOCRINE ORGAN

Adipose tissue produces numerous proteins that act either as local paracrine factors or circulate to modulate both feeding behavior and insulin action. The most well described of these is leptin, which modulates feeding behavior through interaction with specific receptors in the brain. Besides suppressing food intake, leptin also plays a role in modulating glucose and lipid metabolism in the periphery and also regulates energy expenditure. These effects are primarily through the autonomic nervous system, although some actions may be direct. In addition to leptin, the fat cell also expresses resistin, adiponectin, tumor necrosis factor (TNF)-α, interleukin (IL)-6, and likely other proteins that alter the sensitivity of tissues to insulin and may play a role in the pathogenesis of type 2 diabetes.

DEFECTS IN INSULIN SECRETION

Insulin sensitivity is an important factor in determining the magnitude of the insulin response to β-cell stimulation by glucose, its primary secretagogue. When β-cell function is assessed, obese people who are insulin resistant manifest greater responses than lean people. However, the pattern of insulin release is abnormal. The first phase of insulin release is blunted or absent, whereas the second phase is enhanced and prolonged, resulting in overall hyperinsulinemia. The ability of the β-cell to secrete insulin in an oscillatory manner is disrupted, and the ability of the islet to secrete insulin following experimental rises in blood glucose concentrations is blunted. A defect in the normal ratio of proinsulin to insulin is observed with decreased processing of insulin leading to relative increases in proinsulin.

At diagnosis of type 2 diabetes, ~50% of β-cell function has already been lost. With time, further deterioration occurs regardless of dietary, metformin, or sulfonylurea therapy. However, it appears that some stabilization of β-cell function can result from increasing insulin sensitivity by diet, exercise, or treatment with insulin-sensitizing drugs such as the thiazolidinediones. As a result, diabetes appears to be a progressive disorder in which secondary failure of therapeutic interventions is predictable and additional drug therapies are usually required.

In islets, FFAs are important for normal secretion of insulin, whereas excess delivery of FFAs results in a reduction in glucose-stimulated insulin release. The accumulation of long-chain acyl-CoA molecules, leading to disrupted intracellular signaling, oxidative stress, the generation of ceramides, and the accumulation of amyloid protein, have all been proposed to contribute to β-cell dysfunction. Autopsy examinations have demonstrated the association of obesity with an increase in β-cell number, individuals with established type 2 diabetes have about a 50% decrease in β-cell number, and it has been suggested that the decrease in β-cell number is the primary factor in reduction in insulin secretion. Interestingly, decreases are seen in both thin and obese individuals with type 2 diabetes. Although a longitudinal study of β-cell mass is not presently possible, it may be that individuals with diabetes have an intrinsically smaller β-cell mass that predisposed them to the disease.

FACTORS MODULATING INSULIN SECRETION

Incretin hormones (glucagon-like peptide [GLP]-1, gastric inhibitory peptide [GIP]-1, and GIP-2) are released from small intestine endocrine cells following a meal. The proteins act directly on the β-cells to increase their sensitivity to glucose but do not stimulate insulin secretion by themselves. The "incretin" effect of these hormones likely explains the significantly larger secretion of insulin from the β-cell following oral glucose as opposed to that seen following intravenous glucose administration. Some studies suggest that a defect exists in the release and/or response of these hormones in insulin resistance and type 2 diabetes. Pharmacological doses of the native GLP-1 or biologically active analogs, such as extendin-4, can result in a significant potentiation in insulin release in both normal individuals and in those with type 2 diabetes. In contrast, treatment with pharmacological doses of GIP increases insulin secretion only in those without diabetes.

Insulin secretion is also influenced by other gut hormones, including cholecystokinin (CCK), secretin, vasoactive intestinal polypeptide (VIP), and gastrin. What roles these hormones play in blunted insulin secretion in type 2 diabetes remains to be determined, but their effects are believed to be minor.

PHYSIOLOGICAL CONSEQUENCES OF DEFECTIVE INSULIN SECRETION

Regardless of the mechanism, the impairment in insulin secretion in type 2 diabetes following meal ingestion has physiological consequences. When the early phase of insulin secretion is reduced, portal vein insulin concentration remains low after food ingestion and hepatic glucose production is not suppressed. This may be exacerbated by a relative increase in glucagon secretion from islets. Continued output of glucose by the liver plus the glucose entering the circulation from the intestinal tract leads to hyperglycemia. In addition, because of the reduced insulin secretion, glucose uptake by muscle is reduced, accentuating the hyperglycemia. Early in the progression to diabetes, the reduced first-phase insulin secretion is followed by late enhanced insulin secretion. Eventually, the plasma glucose concentration returns to normal, but only at the expense of hyperglycemia and hyperinsulinemia. As the defect in β-cell insulin secretion progresses, even late insulin secretion diminishes. When this occurs, fasting hyperglycemia and overt diabetes develop.

CONCLUSION

Dual defects, insulin resistance and a relative decrease in insulin secretion, are seen in most individuals who have type 2 diabetes and are due to both genetic and environmental factors (Fig. 2.1). Increased insulin resistance is initially compensated for by an increase in insulin secretion, which may be due to increases in islet cell mass and increased production of insulin by individual β-cells. With continued oversupply of nutrients relative to energy expenditure,

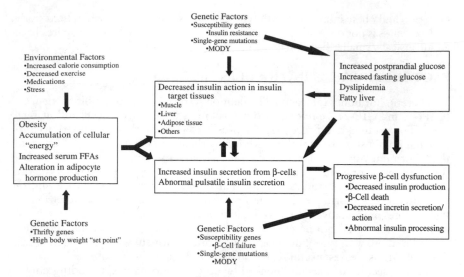

Figure 2.1 Environmental and genetic interactions leading to type 2 diabetes.

the progressive increase in insulin resistance cannot be adequately compensated for by increased insulin secretion, resulting first in impaired glucose tolerance and then diabetes. The cellular mechanisms resulting in muscle, liver, adipose tissue resistance, and β-cell failure may be similar. Alterations in intracellular metabolism resulting from the accumulation of excess energy and manifested by increased intracellular triglyceride levels could provide a unifying pathophysiology. The underlying genetic makeup of the individual dictates whether this prolonged energy imbalance results in hyperglycemia and the associated metabolic disorders associated with type 2 diabetes. Hyperglycemia and dyslipidemia themselves result in additional decreases in insulin action and insulin secretion, reinforcing the established defects in the tissues. Prevention and treatment of insulin resistance and diabetes are initially targeted to limit the positive energy balance and then to modulate the metabolic dysfunction once diabetes is established.

BIBLIOGRAPHY

Boden G: Pathogenesis of type 2 diabetes: insulin resistance. *Endocrinol Metab Clin North Am* 30:801–815, 2001

Boden G, Shulman G: Free fatty acids in obesity and type 2 diabetes: defining their role in the development of insulin resistance and β-cell dysfunction. *Eur J Clin Invest* 32 (Suppl. 3):14–23, 2002

Buchanan TA: Pancreatic beta-cell loss and preservation in type 2 diabetes. *Clin Ther* 25 (Suppl. B):B32–B46, 2003

Kahn SE: The importance of B-cell failure in the development and progression of type 2 diabetes. *J Clin Endocrinol Metab* 86:4047–4058, 2001

Petersen KF, Shulman GI: Pathogenesis of skeletal muscle insulin resistance in type 2 diabetes mellitus. *Am J Cardiol* 90:11G–18G, 2002

Pratley RE, Weyer C: The role of impaired early insulin secretion in the pathogenesis of type II diabetes mellitus. *Diabetologia* 44:929–945, 2001

Tools of Therapy

Highlights

Therapeutic Objectives and Plan

Nutrition
  Body Weight
  Protein
  Fat
  Carbohydrate
  Sugar and Fat Substitutes
  Vitamins and Minerals
  Alcohol

Exercise
  Benefits of Exercise
  Type and Duration of Exercise
  Preexercise Evaluation

Pharmacologic Intervention for Glycemia
  Available Agents
  Selecting an Agent to Begin Treatment
  Primary and Secondary Failure of Treatments
  Starting Insulin Therapy
  Long-Term Combinations of Oral Agents with Insulin
  Adjusting Insulin Dosage in Long-Term Type 2 Diabetes

Assessment of Treatment Efficacy

Office Methods

Patient Monitoring

Highlights
Tools of Therapy

THERAPEUTIC OBJECTIVES AND PLAN

■ Major goals in type 2 diabetes management are
- preventing microvascular and macrovascular complications
- avoiding symptoms related to adverse events of medications and hyperglycemia

■ Specific goals of therapy are to
- eliminate symptoms
- optimize glycemic control
- achieve and maintain reasonable body weight
- achieve and maintain blood pressure control
- achieve and maintain optimal lipid parameters
- identify, prevent, and treat microvascular and macrovascular complications
- achieve optimal overall health and well-being

■ Recommended treatment modalities include
- medical nutrition therapy to improve glucose and lipid parameters and achieve desired body weight
- physical activity to improve glucose control and cardiovascular health
- pharmacologic intervention

■ Individualize therapy based on patient age, comorbidities, lifestyle, financial restrictions, self-management skills learned, and level of patient motivation.

■ Recommendations for metabolic control are found in Table 3.1.

■ Patient education that enhances self-care behaviors is essential for the successful management of type 2 diabetes mellitus.

NUTRITION

■ Medical nutrition therapy is an essential element in the therapeutic plan for patients with type 2 diabetes. For some, nutrition and exercise are the only interventions needed to control the metabolic abnormalities associated with type 2 diabetes, including hyperglycemia, dyslipidemia, and hypertension.

■ Approximately 80–90% of people with type 2 diabetes are obese; thus, weight loss is initially the primary treatment goal. Caloric restriction itself is usually successful in lowering plasma glucose levels even before substantial weight loss is achieved. Approaches to weight reduction are outlined in Overweight.

■ Patients with type 2 diabetes who are of normal weight should eat sufficient calories to maintain that weight and should distribute nutrient intake throughout the day to optimize blood glucose control.

■ Nutrient content of the diet, including fat, protein, carbohydrates, sugar and fat substitutes, and micronutrients, and use of alcohol, must be individualized.

■ Carbohydrates have the greatest impact on postprandial blood glucose response. Setting a carbohydrate goal for meals and snacks is one of the best ways to maximize dietary effectiveness.

EXERCISE

■ Exercise is an essential part of the therapy for the vast majority of patients with type 2 diabetes.

■ Exercise results in improved glycemic control, reduced blood pressure, maintenance or loss of weight, and improvement in dyslipidemia and markers of cardiovascular risk.

■ Individualized daily exercise is important for each patient. Exercise more strenuous than brisk walking requires screening patients at risk for complications and adverse cardiovascular effects.

■ Patients treated with insulin or insulin secretagogues or sulfonylureas may need changes in timing or dose of medication.

PHARMACOLOGIC INTERVENTION FOR GLYCEMIA

■ When a patient is unable to achieve normal or near-normal glucose levels with dietary changes and exercise, despite adequate education and effort, pharmacologic treatment should be implemented.

■ Pharmacologic intervention is an adjunct to and not a substitute for dietary modification and exercise.

■ The choice among antidiabetic agents should be individualized, taking into account patient preferences, comorbidities/contraindications, goals, patient's ability for self-care management, social support, and finances.

■ Oral antidiabetic agents differ from one another in terms of mechanism of action, physiological effect, pharmacokinetics, and metabolism (Tables 3.8 and 3.9).
- Insulin secretagogues (sulfonylureas and glinides) stimulate β-cell insulin secretion.
- The biguanide metformin reduces hepatic glucose overproduction.
- α-Glucosidase inhibitors delay the absorption of carbohydrates from the intestine.
- Thiazolidinediones primarily work in fat and muscle to enhance insulin action.

■ In most patients, a combination of oral agents or oral agents with insulin are required for adequate glycemic control.

■ Insulin therapy augmenting the relative insulin deficiency seen in type 2 diabetes can result in satisfactory control in many patients. Large quantities of insulin may be required because of significant insulin resistance in some patients.

■ Insulin therapy is arguably the most effective and best validated treatment to reduce glucose and risk of complications in diabetes management. It is preferred in the setting of marked (>300 mg/dl [>16.7 mmol/l]) or symptomatic hyperglycemia, in pregnancy, and during hospitalization and is an appropriate choice for many patients with diabetes.

■ The appropriate insulin prescription depends on the amount of β-cell function remaining, whether oral agents are continued, and the daily glucose pattern as determined by self-monitoring of blood glucose (SMBG) among other factors. Some patients with mild to moderate fasting hyperglycemia may be adequately controlled with one injection of intermediate- or long-acting insulin before breakfast or at bedtime. Many patients require a multidose regimen consisting of rapid- or short-acting insulin in combination with either intermediate- or long-acting insulin.

■ Factors that influence the choice of treatments in individual patients are outlined in Selecting an Agent to Begin Treatment. When prescribing a pharmacologic treatment, initially, a low but effective dose should be used, and the dose should be increased on a schedule suited to that agent until the desired glycemic control is achieved, until the maximum effective dose is reached, or until adverse consequences are observed.

■ Some patients maintained on low doses of medications can discontinue the agents and control glucose levels with nutrition and exercise.

■ From 10 to 20% of patients each year experience loss of glycemic control, which may be due to nonadherence, progression of disease, or the development of a superimposed stressful condition. Control of blood glucose can often be restored after secondary failure of a single agent by addition of a second agent with a different mechanism of action.

■ Each individual antidiabetic therapy is in general well tolerated, but each has relative risks and benefits as well as contraindications. There are inadequate head-to-head studies to establish any one therapy as clearly preferred in all patients.

■ Several drugs in common use today can cause hyperglycemia or hypoglycemia (Table 3.11). When possible, these drugs should be avoided.

ASSESSMENT OF TREATMENT EFFICACY

■ The therapeutic response to the treatment of diabetes mellitus is monitored by determining effects on glucose, blood pressure, lipids, and weight as well as signs and symptoms of complications of diabetes.

■ Patients can determine the effects of therapy by SMBG. They can use a daily journal to record food intake, exercise, doses of insulin or oral hypoglycemic agent, symptoms, and results of self-administered blood checks. In individuals with type 2 diabetes, the monitoring of urine ketones is usually not necessary.

■ Physicians monitor the responses to treatment by reviewing with the patient his or her SMBG results as an index of day-to-day control and with assays for glycated hemoglobin, a reflection of degree of glucose control for the preceding 6–12 weeks.

■ Problem solving using SMBG results makes it possible for most patients to achieve near-normal glycemia.

Tools of Therapy

THERAPEUTIC OBJECTIVES AND PLAN

The two major management goals for the patient with type 2 diabetes are to prevent complications and to avoid or alleviate symptoms. Although diabetes is a disease defined on the basis of abnormalities of glucose metabolism, in the setting of type 2 diabetes, it can be argued that aggressive management of blood pressure and lipids, smoking cessation, and antiplatelet therapy are the most important aspects of care given that most patients with diabetes succumb to heart attack or stroke or their consequences. Glucose management is important as it may further reduce cardiovascular risk and clearly lowers the risk of development and progression of diabetic retinopathy, nephropathy, and neuropathy. A summary of recommended targets for adults with diabetes is provided (Table 3.1).

The evidence that long-term glycemic control can prevent or ameliorate the microvascular and neuropathic complications of diabetes comes from a series of clinical trials. The Diabetes Control and Complications Trial (DCCT) demonstrated the beneficial effects of glycemic control in slowing the progression of retinopathy, nephropathy, and neuropathy in type 1 diabetes. The United Kingdom Prospective Diabetes Study (UKPDS) demonstrated in patients with new-onset type 2 diabetes that a more intensive policy of drug therapy with metformin, sulfonylurea, or insulin in addition to lifestyle intervention improved glycemic control and provided for a parallel reduction in the risk of development of combined end points—largely microvascular, with a trend toward reduction in cardiovascular events. In both of these trials, the more intensively treated group exhibited an average glycated hemoglobin A_{1c} (A1C) ~7%; thus, an A1C target of <7% has been adopted as the treatment target for patients with diabetes, because the relative risks and benefits at this level of glycemic control are well established.

The absolute risk of end-stage microvascular complications developing over an intermediate time frame (6–10 years) is small at an A1C ~7%. At A1C levels <7%, the risk of hypoglycemia increases substantially and continues to climb with further lowering of A1C. Thus, it is unclear what the absolute benefit of efforts to achieve A1C targets <7% is, and decisions to pursue lower targets need to be individualized. The UKPDS and the Steno-2 Study (Gaede et al.) demonstrated that intensifying blood pressure, lipid, and glycemic management resulted in substantial reduction in both microvascular and macrovascular complications. A more specific discussion of cardiovascular risk reduction strategies is found in the section on Complications.

Table 3.1 Recommended Metabolic Targets in Adults with Diabetes

Glycemic control	
A1C	<7.0%*
Preprandial plasma glucose	90–130 mg/dl (5.0–7.2 mmol/l)
Postprandial plasma glucose[†]	<180 mg/dl (<10.0 mmol/l)
Blood pressure	<130/80 mmHg
Lipids[‡]	
LDL cholesterol	<100 mg/dl (<2.6 mmol/l)
Triglyceride	<150 mg/dl (<1.7 mmol/l)
HDL cholesterol	>40 mg/dl (<1.1 mmol/l)[§]

Key concepts in setting glycemic goals:

- Goals should be individualized.
- Certain populations (children, pregnant women, and elderly) require special considerations.
- Less intensive glycemic goals may be indicated in patients with severe or frequent hypoglycemia.
- More stringent glycemic goals (i.e., a normal A1C, <6%) may further reduce complications at the cost of increased risk of hypoglycemia (particularly in those with type 1 diabetes).
- Postprandial glucose may be targeted if A1C goals are not met despite reaching preprandial glucose goals.

From American Diabetes Association.
*Referenced to a nondiabetic range of 4.0–6.0% using a DCCT-based assay.
†Postprandial glucose measurements should be made 1–2 h after the beginning of the meal, when levels generally peak in people with diabetes.
‡Current National Cholesterol Education Program Adult Treatment Panel III guidelines suggest that in patients with triglycerides ≥200 mg/dl, the "non-HDL cholesterol" (total cholesterol minus HDL) be utilized. The goal is <130 mg/dl.
§For women, it has been suggested that the HDL goal be increased by 10 mg/dl.

A rational approach to the treatment of elevated blood glucose in patients with type 2 diabetes should include measures that will specifically reverse the underlying pathogenic metabolic disturbances that result in hyperglycemia, insulin resistance, and impaired β-cell function. It is critical to educate patients and their families on self-care practices necessary to manage diabetes. National standards exist for diabetes education programs, and these should be followed (National Standards for Diabetes Self-Management Education, available at www.diabetes.org). As part of this process, a meal plan and exercise program should be developed, pharmacologic therapy should be instituted if necessary, and a monitoring program both at home and in the health care setting needs to be established to assess control. Within this scheme, careful attention to psychosocial influences and/or behavior modification techniques are valuable as outlined in the section on Behavior Change Strategies.

BIBLIOGRAPHY

American Diabetes Association: Standards of medical care in diabetes (Position Statement). *Diabetes Care* 27 (Suppl. 1):S15–S35, 2004

Diabetes Control and Complications Trial Research Group: The effect of intensive treatment of diabetes on the development and progression of long-term complications in insulin-dependent diabetes mellitus. *N Engl J Med* 329:977–986, 1993

Gaede P, Vedel P, Larsen N, Jensen GV, Parving HH, Pedersen O: Multifactorial intervention and cardiovascular disease in patients with type 2 diabetes. *N Engl J Med* 348:383–393, 2003

NCEP Expert Panel on Detection, Evaluation and Treatment of High Blood Cholesterol in Adults: Executive Summary of the Third Report of the National Cholesterol Education Program (NCEP) Expert Panel on Detection, Evaluation and Treatment of High Blood Cholesterol in Adults (Adult Treatment Panel III). *JAMA* 285:2486–2497, 2001

UK Prospective Diabetes Study Group: Intensive blood-glucose control with sulphonylureas or insulin compared with conventional treatment and risk of complications in patients with type 2 diabetes (UKPDS 33). *Lancet* 352:837–853, 1998

UK Prospective Diabetes Study Group: Effect of intensive blood-glucose control with metformin on complications in overweight patients with type 2 diabetes (UKPDS 34). *Lancet* 352:854–865, 1998

NUTRITION

Type 2 diabetes develops due to excessive caloric intake in susceptible individuals. Thus, nutrition therapy is the cornerstone of treatment in type 2 diabetes and should be part of the continuing care of the patient throughout the course of the disease.

Medical nutrition therapy in diabetes is an interactive, collaborative, continuous process of modifying nutrient intake involving the person with diabetes and his or her health care team. It involves

- assessment: evaluating an individual's usual food intake, metabolic status, lifestyle, and readiness to make changes
- goal setting: prioritizing with the patient the areas needing improvement and deciding together what is an achievable and realistic goal
- dietary modification and instruction: teaching the person with diabetes to understand the types and portions of foods to include in a healthy diet, how to read a food label, and the role of carbohydrates in glycemic control so he or she can successfully implement a meal plan that improves metabolic status
- evaluation of successful implementation and follow-up: self-monitoring of blood glucose (SMBG) is necessary to evaluate the effects of diet and exercise on glycemic excursions, and routine glycated hemoglobin (A1C) and serum lipid levels provide feedback on macronutrient intake

In many people with type 2 diabetes, an appropriate combination of nutrition and exercise is the only therapeutic intervention needed to effectively control the metabolic abnormalities associated with this disease. The goals of medical nutrition therapy in type 2 diabetes are to

- maintain near-normal blood glucose levels
- normalize serum lipid levels and blood pressure
- attain and maintain a reasonable body weight
- promote overall health

Because of the heterogeneous nature of type 2 diabetes, there is no single prescription for dietary modification that will achieve these goals in all patients. The meal plan must be individualized. Diversity in insulin secretion capacity and insulin resistance, as well as personal characteristics related to cultural and social characteristics, lifestyle, age, body weight, and medication regimen, influence strategies chosen to achieve the nutrition goals. Eating habits, attitude, and learning abilities also influence the ability to achieve nutrition goals. Several obstacles to dietary adherence have been identified and should be considered in the dietary assessment and evaluation plan (Table 3.2).

Guidelines for nutritional intervention in individuals with diabetes have been developed that consider the heterogeneity of diabetes (Table 3.3). The success of a particular dietary intervention is evaluated via metabolic parameters, as well as quality of life and body weight. Failure of one intervention strategy may be corrected by using another.

Table 3.2 Obstacles to Dietary Adherence for Adults with Diabetes

- Resisting temptation: social events, special foods, cues, or cravings trigger noncompliance
- Eating out: difficult to control portions and ingredients
- Feeling deprived: regret not being able to eat like people without diabetes
- Negative emotions: attempt to cope by overeating
- Temptation to relapse: feeling of wanting to give up or take a vacation
- Planning/priorities: it takes too much time to prepare foods on the meal plan; other things get in the way
- Family/friends: support is not offered and/or positive behaviors not modeled

Adapted from Schlundt et al.

BODY WEIGHT

Body mass index (BMI) is used as a practical definition of body weight relative to health risk. It defines overweight and obesity calculated as weight in kilograms divided by the square of height in meters, thus kg/m². The U.S. Dietary Guidelines for Americans have defined a healthy weight as BMI 19–24.9. A BMI calculator is available at http://www.cdc.gov/nccdphp/dnpa/bmi/calc-bmi.htm. BMI ≥25 has been generally accepted as a definition of overweight, and BMI ≥30 is indicative of obesity. Because body weight profoundly influences insulin resistance, insulin requirements, and subsequent blood glucose control, an appropriate daily caloric intake is integral to the nutrition plan in type 2 diabetes. However, caloric intake may not require modification if BMI is normal or an individual is unwilling or unable to restrict intake.

Valuable steps to include in a weight loss program are obtaining a body weight history and working with the patient to create a diet log, a 24-h diet recall, or a 3-day diet history to use in estimating usual daily caloric intake and eating patterns.

Normal Weight

Approximately 10–20% of people with type 2 diabetes have normal BMI and may therefore not need their caloric intake modified. Asian Americans in particular seem to have a higher risk of diabetes at moderate BMIs. For normal-weight individuals, the focus of the nutrition plan can be on modifying carbohydrate content of the diet, and the distribution of carbohydrate between meals and snacks becomes the primary intervention.

The elderly or those individuals with additional medical problems that increase metabolic needs (e.g., wound healing, neuropathy, gastrointestinal disturbances) may need to increase caloric intake to provide enough calories, protein, vitamins, and minerals to promote healing and anabolic processes.

Carbohydrates have the greatest impact on postprandial blood glucose response. Setting a carbohydrate goal for meals and snacks is one of the best ways to maximize dietary effectiveness. Patients can be taught to increase or decrease

Table 3.3 Nutrition Goals, Principles, and Recommendations

- **Calories**
  - Sufficient to attain and/or maintain a reasonable body weight for adults, normal growth and development for children and adolescents, and adequate nutrition during pregnancy and lactation
- **Protein**
  - 10–20% of daily calories
  - No more than 0.8 g/kg body weight/day in people with evidence of nephropathy
- **Fat**
  - Saturated fat <10% of daily calories, <7% with elevated LDL cholesterol
  - Polyunsaturated fat up to 10% of total calories
  - Remaining total fat varies with treatment goals
    - □ ~30%—normal weight and lipids
    - □ <30%—obese, elevated LDL cholesterol
    - □ ≤40%—elevated triglycerides unresponsive to fat restriction and weight loss
    - □ Predominately monounsaturated fat
- **Cholesterol**
  - <300 mg/day
- **Carbohydrate**
  - Difference after protein and fat goals have been met
  - Percentage varies with treatment goals
- **Sweeteners**
  - Sucrose need not be restricted, must be substituted as carbohydrate
  - Nutritive sweeteners have no advantage over sucrose and must be substituted as carbohydrate
  - Nonnutritive sweeteners approved by the FDA are safe to consume
- **Fiber**
  - 20–35 g/day
- **Sodium**
  - <3,000 mg/day
  - <2,400 mg/day in mild to moderate hypertension
- **Alcohol**
  - Moderate usage, i.e., up to 2 servings of alcohol daily in men and up to 1 daily in women
- **Vitamins and Minerals**
  - Same as the general population

Goals must always be individualized.

carbohydrate intake per meal and/or snack to yield optimal blood glucose results. If they use rapid- or short-acting insulin, they may be able to adjust insulin dose to compensate for changes in carbohydrate intake by employing an insulin-to-carbohydrate ratio.

The quality and quantity of fats in the diet can affect lipid levels. Saturated fats, *trans* saturated fats, and cholesterol intake may increase circulating atherogenic lipid particles, particularly LDL cholesterol and the triglyceride-rich VLDL cholesterol and remnant particles. Monounsaturated fats often have a beneficial effect on these lipid particles. Intake and proportion of calories from fat should be dictated by the level of dyslipidemia as well as the level of carbohydrate that optimizes blood glucose.

Diets with varying quantity and sources of carbohydrate, lipids, and proteins have been widely touted in the lay and medical press. Many individuals with type 2 diabetes are presently experimenting with these diets. Because long-term studies have not proven the relative risks and benefits of each, recommending initiation or continuation of these diets should be done on an individual basis, considering the resulting weight loss may provide a benefit to overall health.

Overweight

Approximately 80–90% of people with type 2 diabetes are obese; thus, weight loss is initially the primary treatment goal. Calorie restriction itself may be responsible for improved glucose tolerance, because the loss of as little as 5–10% of body weight improves insulin sensitivity and glucose uptake, reduces insulin secretory requirements, and decreases hepatic glucose production. Weight loss may be most beneficial early in the diagnosis of type 2 diabetes when insulin secretion is most robust.

Weight reduction can be accomplished by a combination of modest caloric restriction, physical activity, behavior modification of eating habits, and psychosocial support. Most individuals will regain lost weight. It has been suggested that such fluctuations in weight are unhealthy for modestly overweight individuals, but little scientific evidence substantiates this concern. On the other hand, the effects of weight gain of as little as 20 lb after age 18 on chronic disease and health are becoming increasingly evident. Body fat distributed above the waist increases the risk of developing diabetes, cardiovascular disease, and hypertension. A waist-to-hip ratio >1.0 or waist ≥40 inches (102 cm) in men and waist-to-hip ratio >0.8 or waist ≥35 inches (88 cm) in women increases risk for cardiovascular mortality.

Because of the psychological and physiological impact of "dieting," obese individuals should be encouraged to attain a reasonable body weight as determined by BMI. Note that reasonable weight is defined as the weight an individual and health care provider acknowledge as achievable and maintainable, in both the short and long term. This may not be the same as the defined desirable or ideal BMI (i.e., <25).

A beneficial weight-loss goal is ~2 BMI units or approximately 8–16 lb initially. The U.S. Dietary Guidelines for Americans endorse small weight losses of 0.5–1.0 lb/week. Not only does an overall weight loss of 5–10 lb improve glucose tolerance, it also reduces blood pressure and serum lipid levels. Because weight gain in an overweight individual is medically detrimental, and losing weight and keeping it off is extremely difficult, preventing weight gain should be given the same importance as weight loss in an obese individual. A healthy diet plan of moderation combined with daily physical activity is the primary intervention in type 2 diabetes.

A 3,500-kcal deficit will produce a loss of 1 lb of body fat. Daily calorie intake should be evaluated with a diet history and adjusted to produce a modest deficit. Generally, a decrease of 500 calories/day is needed to produce a 1-lb loss of fat/week. This can vary, however, based on the individual and his or her willingness to restrict intake and/or increase activity. Regular exercise enhances weight loss and is identified as a predictor for successful weight maintenance.

Alternative approaches for calorie restriction are possible with individuals who are seriously overweight. Restrictive very-low-calorie diets (600–800 kcal/day) are sometimes used in type 2 diabetes. This medically supervised approach generally involves a liquid formula, but may be accomplished with high-quality lean protein sources (1.5 g/kg body weight/day) with vitamin and mineral supplementation. Weight loss is rapid (3–5 lb/week), and hyperglycemia generally improves within 24 h of implementation. Near-maximum blood glucose improvement is achieved within 10 days of initiating this regimen. However, this approach should be restricted to individuals who are at least 30% above desirable weight (BMI >30). For some, using this regimen for as short a period as 2–12 week can provide the psychological motivation needed to encourage dietary adherence and may, in fact, improve blood glucose control enough to minimize the need for pharmacological therapy. Alternating a very-low-calorie dietary regimen with a modest caloric reduction has been used successfully in some studies, as has a weekly "day of fasting," and may be a potential alternative for some individuals. Because a restriction of <1,200 calories for women and <1,500 calories for men is difficult to adhere to and can be nutritionally inadequate, most individuals will be more successful if they reduce usual daily intake by 250 calories and increase daily activity by 250 calories. If the diet history is unreliable, approximate daily calorie intake can be estimated by multiplying actual weight in pounds by a factor of 10–15 (the factor decreases with age and decreasing physical activity level).

Pharmacotherapy for the treatment of obesity is considered safe and modestly effective in high-risk obese individuals, including those with type 2 diabetes. Each medication has its benefits and risks and should be prescribed only with close medical supervision. Most people will regain the lost weight once the medication is stopped. Therefore, research into the potential long-term use of these drugs is ongoing.

Surgical interventions have been successful in people with a BMI >40. A significant and sustained weight loss can be achieved with banding and bypass procedures in most patients but can be associated with a number of side effects such as infection, liver disease, dumping syndrome, or even death. Like pharmacotherapy, surgery is only an adjunct to diet and exercise.

People with type 2 diabetes who take oral hypoglycemic agents or insulin may require a decrease or discontinuation of the medication as calorie or carbohydrate restriction is implemented and as weight loss progresses. This may be a gradual reduction with a modestly hypocaloric diet or a rapid reduction (>50%) with a very-low-calorie diet. In addition, some studies suggest that excessive doses of insulin or hypoglycemic agents may lead to hunger and overeating, which is counterproductive in obesity.

The results of SMBG provide the necessary feedback to make adjustments in nutrition and medication therapy. Frequent follow-up with a dietitian provides problem-solving techniques and encouragement and supports the weight-loss efforts (see Chapter 6, Behavior Change Strategies). This can be done individually or in groups. Appropriate referrals to local hospital programs or other weight-loss programs with qualified staff are useful.

PROTEIN

The recommendation for protein intake in type 2 diabetes is the U.S. recommended dietary allowance (RDA) of 0.8 g/kg body weight/day for adults. Typically, larger amounts are consumed in Western diets (1.2–2.0 g/kg body weight/day). Thus, protein accounts for ~12–20% or more of typical total calorie consumption. Because excessive protein consumption may aggravate glomerular hyperfiltration, the pathophysiologic mechanism for the development and progression of renal insufficiency, 0.8–1.0 g/kg body weight/day, may represent an optimal goal in those with albuminuria and renal insufficiency. This goal is reflected in the USDA Food Guide Pyramid recommendation of 5–7 oz lean protein daily. Accomplishing this goal gradually over several months or even years may be necessary because it represents a major alteration in attitude toward protein in the diet. Meat, fish, and poultry are limited to 3–5 oz/day on a 0.8 g/kg regimen.

More severe restriction (0.6 g/kg body weight/day) has been suggested to reduce proteinuria and slow the progression of renal failure in patients who exhibit some renal insufficiency. Compliance with such a regimen is difficult, and studies have suggested that muscle wasting and loss of total-body protein can result. Therefore, individuals with diabetes should not consume <0.8 g/kg body weight/day protein. Increasing evidence suggests that not all proteins have the same effect on the kidneys. Vegetable protein has been shown to result in a lower glomerular filtration rate and renal plasma flow—suggestive of less stress on the kidney than certain animal proteins (e.g., beef). There is limited evidence demonstrating that individuals with type 2 diabetes with lack of insulin secretion to glucose stimuli continue to secrete insulin in response to protein ingestion (specifically, certain amino acids). The glycemic effect of adding or subtracting protein from a given meal or snack can be evaluated with SMBG.

FAT

With protein accounting for 10–20% of total calories, remaining calories will be derived from a combination of fat and carbohydrate. The proportion derived from either depends on the desired medical outcome for each individual patient. Lipid abnormalities common in type 2 diabetes are influenced by carbohydrate and fat content of the diet as well as by body weight, genetics, physical activity, and glycemic control. Hypertriglyceridemia and low HDL cholesterol are the most common lipid abnormalities in type 2 diabetes. This dyslipidemia has been shown to be a significant risk factor for cardiovascular disease in people with and without diabetes.

High-carbohydrate low-fat diets, although recommended by many health organizations and nutrition experts to reduce total and LDL cholesterol, have been shown to increase postprandial blood glucose and triglyceride levels, elevate fasting triglyceride levels, and decrease HDL cholesterol levels in insulin-resistant people, including those with type 2 diabetes. This has sparked concern over the wisdom of recommending a low-fat diet in insulin-resistant type 2 diabetes. Several investigators have shown improved lipid levels and blood glucose control in both short- and intermediate-term studies in which total fat intake approaches 45% of calories and carbohydrate intake is as low as 40% of calories.

Because saturated fat intake should comprise fewer than 10% of total calories and polyunsaturated fats up to 10%, any increase in fat calories should come from monounsaturated fats. Indeed, studies comparing low-fat with low-carbohydrate diets in type 2 diabetes have used monounsaturated fat in amounts up to 25% of

Table 3.4 Common Sources of Monounsaturated Fat

Type of Fat	Percentage of Total Lipid
Vegetable	
Canola (rapeseed)	66
Olive	74
Peanut	46
Soybean	23
Animal	
Beef	43
Butter	29
Chicken/turkey	39/32
Salmon	35

Adapted from Agriculture Handbook, No. 8 Series, U.S. Department of Agriculture, Human Information Service.

calories. Major sources of monounsaturated fat include olive, canola, and peanut oils (Table 3.4). However, animal fat, such as that found in beef, pork, and poultry, is nearly one-third monounsaturated fat. Substituting olive and canola oils for other vegetable oils and margarines can be augmented by adding nuts, olives, and avocado to meals and snacks.

Concern that increasing fat intake could potentially lead to weight gain has proved unfounded, at least in the setting of carbohydrate restriction, as a review of controlled clinical studies using high–monounsaturated fat low-carbohydrate diets demonstrates. However, both short- and intermediate-term weight loss studies demonstrate that similar or greater weight loss is associated with lower-carbohydrate diet approaches. Reducing fat or carbohydrate intake in obese individuals will not necessarily lead to reduced calories; weight loss will only occur if calories are restricted, and approaches that limit fat and particularly highly processed and easily digestible carbohydrates are most appropriate. A low-fat diet without weight loss may or may not result in improved lipid levels in an obese person with type 2 diabetes.

Obese people with diabetes should be given substantial time (weeks to months) on a individualized diet plan that reduces fat and carbohydrate intake with a goal of reducing calories. If metabolic parameters such as serum lipids and blood glucose control do not improve, consider a moderate fat increase using monounsaturated fats with a simultaneous further reduction in carbohydrate intake. Close follow-up and monitoring of metabolic parameters should guide further dietary adjustments.

Saturated fats should make up <10% total calories because of their dramatic effect on serum total and LDL cholesterol levels. Currently, adults in the U.S. consume ~13% total calories from saturated fat. Saturated fatty acids have been shown to be twice as potent in raising plasma cholesterol as polyunsaturated fats are in lowering them. Saturated fatty acids are predominately found in animal products. Coconut and palm oils are highly saturated vegetable oils used in baked products, such as cookies and crackers. Whole-milk dairy products and baked goods contribute more to the saturated fat content of the U.S. diet than do meat and meat products. Thus, the most effective way to reduce saturated fat content of the diet is to substitute low-fat milk products, limit meat to lean cuts and reasonable portions, and use baked products made with vegetable oils that have not been hydrogenated.

Cholesterol intake should be limited to <300 mg/day. All animal products, including meat, poultry, eggs, cheese, full-fat dairy products, and shellfish, contain cholesterol. Consuming low-fat dairy products and lean cuts of meat and limiting eggs to ~4/week are the most substantial ways to reduce dietary cholesterol intake. Note that although decreasing cholesterol intake reduces serum cholesterol levels, quantitatively, its effect is less than that of lowering saturated fat. The beneficial effect of substituting poultry and fish for red meat is primarily due to the reduced saturated fat content of poultry and fish, because the cholesterol content may be similar. The level of serum cholesterol reduction one can expect from dietary reduction of fat and cholesterol will vary with the individual.

Polyunsaturated vegetable fats are liquid at room temperature but can be hydrogenated to yield a more solid product, such as margarine or shortening. In the process, *trans* fatty acids, which have proven to be as atherogenic as saturated fats in controlled clinical trials, are created. Epidemiological studies have also found an association between the *trans* fatty acid content of the diet and an increased risk of cardiovascular disease. Vegetable oils and soft margarines are preferred polyunsaturated fat sources.

Fish oil contains polyunsaturated fatty acids in the form of ω-3 fatty acids. The ω-3 fatty acids have a beneficial effect on cardiovascular disease risk by reducing serum triglycerides and decreasing platelet aggregation. Consuming 8 oz fish each week has been suggested as an effective way to increase ω-3 fatty acid intake. Salmon, albacore tuna, lake trout, and herring are excellent sources.

CARBOHYDRATE

The amount and type of carbohydrate that should be included in the diet of a person with type 2 diabetes should be individualized and, as with fat and protein, be driven by the predominant metabolic abnormality the patient seeks to improve. If LDL and total cholesterol are elevated, then the initial diet plan should restrict fat to ≤30%. This would result in ~50–60% of calories being derived from carbohydrate. The clinician should then carefully evaluate daily blood glucose levels and A1C values along with their impact on serum triglycerides and cholesterol to determine whether this plan is achieving the desired medical outcomes. If not, a gradual decrease in carbohydrate may be warranted with a subsequent increase in fat, predominantly monounsaturated fat. The USDA Food Guide Pyramid is a good source for recommending carbohydrate choices for individuals with type 2 diabetes. Its emphasis on whole grains, fruits, and vegetables supplies necessary fiber, vitamins, minerals, and antioxidants to the meal plan. The key is to also teach patients the serving sizes listed from each of the food groups.

Clinical research investigating the impact of carbohydrate-containing foods on blood glucose response has shown that some differences among carbohydrates do exist. Research has demonstrated that the longer chains of glucose molecules present in carbohydrates, such as starches, do not necessarily yield a flatter blood glucose response curve than the shorter-chain carbohydrates found in sugars. When equal amounts of carbohydrate are compared, no significant difference in glycemic response is seen. However, factors such as processing, preparation, and rate of digestion affect the glycemic response of a specific food.

Clinically, the most important determinant of glycemic response to a meal is the total carbohydrate content. Fat and protein contribute little to blood glucose response other than slowing the rate of digestion and absorption of carbohydrate. As a result, once the total amount of carbohydrate to be included in the diet is determined, carbohydrate should be distributed between meals and snacks in a pattern than yields the optimal blood glucose responses. Blood glucose testing is crucial in evaluating carbohydrate distribution. Patients requiring insulin can adjust short-acting insulin doses to changing carbohydrate consumption. Testing postprandial glucose levels can help guide the patient in adjusting insulin doses in response to particular carbohydrate meals.

Fiber is a nondigestible form of carbohydrate that contributes bulk to the diet and appears to slow down the digestion and absorption of carbohydrate. Soluble fiber, such as that found in oat bran and legumes, can blunt postprandial blood glucose responses and reduce serum cholesterol levels. Nonsoluble fiber from wheat bran and many fruits and vegetables has little impact on reducing blood glucose or serum cholesterol, but it is necessary for optimal gastrointestinal function. People with diabetes should consume a daily amount of fiber that meets or exceeds the USDA recommendation of 25 g/day.

Sugar restriction is no longer the primary focus of diet therapy in diabetes. Clinical research has not found sugar-containing foods to be detrimental to blood glucose control when substituted gram for gram for other carbohydrates in the diets of people with diabetes. Individuals with diabetes can be instructed how to substitute sugary foods using carbohydrate-counting plans or the exchange system. Obese individuals need to be cautioned that high-sugar foods, such as cookies, pastries, and ice creams, are also high in fat and calories. Portion control and understanding how to read food labels is crucial to success.

The glycemic index is a classification of foods based on their blood glucose–raising potential when studied as single-source meals. Low–glycemic index foods raise glucose less after consumption than high–glycemic index foods. The most appropriate use of these concepts is as supplementary to a comprehensive nutrition plan. Some low–glycemic index foods are poor choices for regular consumption in the setting of diabetes because they are high in fat and relatively devoid of other essential nutrients (e.g., chocolate). Some high–glycemic index foods may be good choices for regular consumption as they are low in calories and full of other nutrients (e.g., carrots). Finally, in some situations, high–glycemic index foods may be appropriate due simply to their convenience and benefits versus other acceptable choices to an individual person in a given situation (e.g., cereal and skim milk versus a bacon, egg, and cheese croissant).

SUGAR AND FAT SUBSTITUTES

Sorbitol, mannitol, and fructose are commonly used sweeteners that have a lower glycemic effect than either glucose or sucrose (table sugar). Fructose contains the same amount of calories as glucose and sucrose (4 kcal/g); thus, it cannot be used ad libitum, particularly in the hypocaloric diet. The sugar alcohols sorbitol and mannitol have only 2–3 kcal/g, but they are often found in products when extra fat has been added. They may cause gastrointestinal distress, such as bloating and diarrhea, when >30 g/day are consumed (10–15 hard candies). Foods containing these sugars must be accounted for in the meal plan.

Noncaloric sweeteners such as acesulfame K, aspartame, neotame, saccharin, and sucralose are >200 times sweeter than sugar. Their use as tabletop sweeteners and in soft drinks is beneficial in diabetes because they contribute no calories or carbohydrates. However, they may be used in foods that contain other sources of carbohydrates and calories, such as ice cream, cookies, and puddings. These foods need to be worked into the meal plan appropriately.

Currently available fat substitutes are derived primarily from carbohydrate or protein. This reduces their caloric value from 9 to 4 kcal/g. However, the use of fat substitutes in foods such as yogurt, ice cream, and salad dressings increases the carbohydrate content of the products above their usual level. Individuals should be advised to consider the carbohydrate level when using such foods.

Fat substitutes such as olestra are made from fat that has been modified to be totally nondigestible and therefore not absorbed. As a result, olestra adds no fat or fat calories to products. It can also produce gastrointestinal distress and occasionally is associated with deficiencies in fat-soluble vitamins. Sugar- and fat-modified foods may be beneficial to people with diabetes by assisting them to reduce their fat, carbohydrate, and calorie intake. However, they are not necessary for a healthy diet and should only be suggested as alternatives.

VITAMINS AND MINERALS

There is no evidence for an increased need for vitamins or minerals in diabetes above the current RDA. Antioxidants, such as β-carotene, vitamin E, and vitamin C, have been suggested to reduce risk of cardiovascular disease, cancer, and cataracts in the general population. Unfortunately, there have been no long-term controlled clinical studies, particularly in people with diabetes, that have shown benefit on the incidence or progression of any of these diseases from antioxidant supplement consumption.

A deficiency of chromium has been implicated in causing insulin resistance. However, a role for chromium supplementation in preventing and treating type 2 diabetes has not been supported by randomized clinical trials. In animal models, high doses of chromium potentiates insulin action, and it is possible that chromium supplementation may be of value in chromium-deficient individuals; however, there is no useful way to evaluate deficiency. Moreover, the long-term effects of chromium supplementation are unknown. Whole-grain products, nuts, and seeds and protein-rich foods are the best sources of chromium, but these can realistically provide only about 50 μg/day.

In a prospective, double-blind, randomized trial, a combination of folic acid (1 mg), vitamin B12 (400 μg), and pyridoxine (10 mg) was shown to reduce homocysteine levels as well as the need for revascularization and rates of restenosis during 6 months of treatment after successful coronary angioplasty. Although about 25% of the patients in this small study had diabetes, no subgroup analysis was provided. Nevertheless, this warrants consideration of B vitamin supplementation in patients with known coronary artery disease and/or hyperhomocysteinemia. This can be easily achieved by the consumption of a multivitamin tablet daily.

Another small randomized, controlled trial demonstrated that multivitamin and mineral supplements reduced the incidence of participant-reported infection and related absenteeism among patients with type 2 diabetes mellitus. A related finding was the high prevalence of subclinical micronutrient deficiency in this rather unselected population.

Sodium recommendations for people with diabetes are no more restrictive than for the general population. For people with mild to moderate hypertension, ≤2,400 mg/day of sodium is recommended. Severe sodium restriction seems to be less valuable than weight loss in controlling hypertension in obese people with type 2 diabetes.

ALCOHOL

Abstinence from alcohol is not necessary for patients with diabetes mellitus. In most cases, moderate amounts of alcohol (up to two servings daily for men and one serving daily for nonpregnant women), as recommended for the general population, are allowable in diabetes. Recent studies in the general population have shown reduced cardiovascular disease mortality to be associated with moderate alcohol consumption. Obviously, alcohol consumption is not recommended for people with conditions such as pregnancy, alcoholism, cirrhosis of the liver, and symptomatic neuropathy.

Before a patient may include alcohol in his or her eating plan, the potential problems associated with alcohol consumption should be considered, e.g., alcohol consumption by a person who is fasting (>5 h) or undernourished may lead to hypoglycemia. This can be a serious problem in patients taking insulin or an oral hypoglycemic agent who skip meals. A patient's ability to follow the prescribed management plan will be impaired if he or she is intoxicated. Additionally, alcohol ingestion may be associated with significant elevations in fasting and postprandial plasma triglyceride levels in people with hypertriglyceridemia.

BIBLIOGRAPHY

American Diabetes Association: Nutrition principles and recommendations in diabetes (Position Statement). *Diabetes Care* 27 (Suppl. 1):S36–S46, 2004

Barringer TA, Kirk JK, Santaniello AC, Foley KL, Michielutte R: Effect of a multivitamin and mineral supplement on infection and quality of life: a randomized, double-blind, placebo-controlled trial. *Ann Intern Med* 138:365–371, 2003

Brand-Miller J, Hayne S, Petocz P, Colagiuri S: Low–glycemic index diets in the management of diabetes: a meta-analysis of randomized controlled trials. *Diabetes Care* 26:2261–2267, 2003

DCCT Research Group: Expanded role of the dietitian in the Diabetes Control and Complications Trial: implications for clinical practice. *J Am Diet Assoc* 93:758–764, 767, 1993

Franz MJ, Bantle JP, Beebe CA, Brunzell JD, Chiasson J-L, Garg A, Holzmeister LA, Hoogwerf B, Mayer-Davis E, Mooradian AD, Purnell JQ, Wheeler M: Evidence-based nutrition principles and recommendations for the treatment and prevention of diabetes and related complications (Technical Review). *Diabetes Care* 25:148–198, 2002

Mooridian AD, Failla M, Hoogwerf B, Maryniuk M, Wylie-Rosett J: Selected vitamins and minerals in diabetes. *Diabetes Care* 17:464–479, 1994

Schlundt DG, Rea MR, Kline SS, Pichert JW: Situational obstacles to dietary adherence for adults with diabetes. *J Am Diet Assoc* 94:874–876, 1994

Schnyder G, Roffi M, Pin R, Flammer Y, Lange H, Eberli FR, Meier B, Turi ZG, Hess OM: Decreased rate of coronary restenosis after lowering of plasma homocysteine levels. *N Engl J Med* 345:1593–1600, 2001

U.S. Department of Agriculture: *The Food Guide Pyramid*. Hyattsville, MD, Human Nutrition Information Service, 1992

Yeh GY, Eisenberg DM, Kaptchuk TJ, Phillips RS: Systematic review of herbs and dietary supplements for glycemic control in diabetes. *Diabetes Care* 26:1277–1294, 2003

EXERCISE

The adoption of a sedentary lifestyle is a clear factor in the development of type 2 diabetes. The accumulation of excess energy stores in skeletal muscle in the form of glycogen and triglyceride leads to insulin resistance. Exercise has two effects that improve the metabolic state. Acutely, contraction of skeletal muscle results in the translocation of glucose transporters to the plasma membrane and increases glucose uptake. This acute effect of exercise may be mediated by AMP-dependent protein kinase (AMPK). AMPK is thought to be a sensor of intracellular energy stores and is activated by increases in intracellular AMP. With prolonged exercise training, there is a shift in the dose-response curve for insulin reflecting an increase in insulin sensitivity. The effect of exercise training to increase insulin sensitivity is related to upregulation of glucose transporter number, changes in capillary density, and increases in the number of glycolytic (type IIa) fibers, which have an increased capacity for oxidative metabolism. The latter may be of particular importance, because studies have suggested that individuals with type 2 diabetes have a decrease in mitochondrial oxidation. A decrease in intrinsic oxidative capacity of skeletal muscle has also been found in offspring of individuals with type 2 diabetes who have normal glucose tolerance, which suggests that this may form part of the genetic predisposition to the disease and is a reason why regular exercise, which increases oxidative capacity, contributes to diabetes prevention.

BENEFITS OF EXERCISE

The clinical benefits of exercise in individuals with diabetes include improvement in glycemic control, reduction in blood pressure, maintenance or improvement in body weight, and improvement in dyslipidemia and markers of cardiovascular risk. Other potential benefits are improved insulin sensitivity resulting in a reduction in the progression of β-cell failure, increased vascular reactivity, reduction in arthritis symptoms, reduction in risk of osteoporosis, and improvements in psychological well-being. Finally, three trials have documented that lifestyle modifications that include a regular exercise regimen delay or prevent type 2 diabetes.

Studies have demonstrated that regular aerobic physical activity results in improvements in insulin sensitivity and glycemic control. In some studies, a 50–100% increase in insulin sensitivity has been demonstrated. A1C levels can be reduced by 10–20% of baseline (average of reduction 0.66%), with a greater efficacy in patients with early, uncomplicated type 2 diabetes and those with the highest BMIs. The effects are related to the duration and intensity of exercise, but a clear dose-response effect is not apparent. Exercise-induced enhanced sensitivity to insulin occurs without changes in body weight.

Effect on Markers for Cardiovascular Disease

Although no prospective studies have demonstrated an effect of exercise on age-adjusted risk of cardiovascular events, there appear to be beneficial effects on numerous markers associated with increased risk for cardiovascular disease. Intervention studies have shown that blood pressure is improved by 4.9–6.0/3.7–5.0 mmHg in hypertensive individuals performing variable exercise regimens. This reduction is unrelated to the frequency or intensity of exercise, suggesting that all forms are effective. The effect of exercise on dyslipidemia is mixed. Regular physical activity is consistently effective in reducing levels of total and triglyceride-rich VLDL cholesterol. However, effects on levels of LDL and HDL cholesterol are inconsistent.

Exercise has also been associated with improvements in inflammatory markers, including C-reactive peptide and plasminogen activator inhibitor-1 levels. However, there is no clear consensus on whether physical training results in improved fibrinolytic activity in these patients.

Effect on Body Weight

Increased physical activity can play an important part in weight-reduction programs. Exercise has been identified as the strongest predictor for long-term maintenance of lost weight when used with an appropriate calorie-controlled diet. This information comes from the National Weight Control Registry, in which individuals who have successfully maintained weight loss long term (>1 year) self-report expending an average of 400 calories/day exercising. Some studies have suggested that aerobic exercise decreases abdominal (central) adiposity, which could have a significant effect on metabolic abnormalities. Acute exercise decreases appetite, but this effect appears to be short lived.

TYPE AND DURATION OF EXERCISE

The 1996 Surgeon General's Report on Physical Activity and Health concluded that regular, moderate physical activity offers substantial benefits in health and well-being for the vast majority of Americans who are not physically active. That report defines moderate physical activity as using 150 calories/day, or 1,000 calories/week. To achieve this level of exercise, it is recommended that an otherwise healthy individual sustain 30–40 min of exercise at 50–80% of target heart rate on a daily or near-daily basis. Unless there are contraindications, this exercise intensity and duration is the minimal goal for individuals with type 2 diabetes. Even sedentary individuals can begin a routine of brisk walking. Studies also suggest that resistance training with weights or other resistance devices has a beneficial effect on glucose metabolism and results in increased oxidative fiber types.

In the absence of complications, patients with type 2 diabetes treated by diet alone can exercise in the same manner as people without diabetes. Supplementary food before, during, or after activity is unnecessary, because hypoglycemia is not a risk. However, individuals with type 2 diabetes treated with hypoglycemic agents (insulin, sulfonylureas), especially at the initiation of an exercise program, need to be aware of the insulin-sensitizing effect of exercise and its potential to cause hypoglycemia. Hypoglycemia can occur during or as much as 12–24 h after the exercise session. Records of blood glucose monitoring can guide medication adjustments to prevent exercise-induced hypoglycemia. The dosage of hypoglycemic agents may need to be decreased on days during which exercise is performed, an appropriate alternative to increasing food intake. Finally, it is recommended that all individuals who have diabetes should carry a diabetes identification card or medical alert jewelry.

PREEXERCISE EVALUATION

As with any therapy, exercise regimens should be individualized and monitored for salutary and adverse effects. Specific precautions need to be taken in some individuals to ensure benefit and minimize risk.

Before beginning any program more strenuous than brisk walking, the patient should be evaluated for

- glycemic control
- cardiovascular risks: blood pressure, peripheral pulses, bruits, blood lipids
- neurologic dysfunction including peripheral and autonomic neuropathy
- dilated fundoscopic examination, especially if proliferative retinopathy is present or suspected

A monitored exercise stress test should be performed in individuals who are at elevated risk of cardiovascular disease (Table 3.5).

Special precautions should be taken when a patient requires or uses drugs that may make him or her more susceptible to exercise-induced hypoglycemia. For example, alcohol and very high doses of salicylates should be avoided because they may themselves produce hypoglycemia and can augment any hypoglycemic effect of drug and exercise. The β-adrenergic–blocking agents may prevent the rapid hepatic glyconeolytic responses that normally correct hypoglycemia.

Patients with complications of diabetes need specific counseling on the type and duration of exercise. For example, individuals with gastroparesis are at risk for significant hypoglycemia if exercise follows a meal that is slowly absorbed. Significantly obese patients should avoid exercise that can increase the risk of joint or ligament injury, such as running. Swimming is a highly beneficial exercise that has the least impact on the lower extremities. Specific precautions are outlined in Table 3.6.

Ischemic heart disease can be present without chest pain. Autonomic neuropathy and β-blockers may interfere with maximal heart rate and exercise performance. This is in addition to the already observed 15–20% lower age-matched maximal heart rate found in people with type 2 diabetes. Lower target heart rates

Table 3.5 Guidelines for Stress Testing Before Initiating an Exercise Program

- Age >40 yr
- Age >35 yr and
  - Diabetes >10 yr duration
  - Any additional risk factor for coronary artery disease: hypertension, dyslipidemia, cigarette smoking
  - Presence of microvascular disease: proliferative retinopathy or nephropathy, including microalbuminuria
- Any of the following, regardless of age:
  - Known or suspected coronary artery disease, cerebrovascular disease, and/or peripheral vascular disease
  - Autonomic neuropathy
  - Renal failure

Table 3.6 Precautions for Patients with Medical Complications

- Insensitive feet or peripheral vascular insufficiency
  - Avoid running
  - Choose walking, cycling, or swimming
  - Emphasize proper footwear
- Untreated or recently treated proliferative retinopathy: avoid exercises associated with
  - Increased intra-abdominal pressure
  - Valsalva-like maneuvers
  - Rapid head movements
  - Eye trauma
- Hypertension and/or retinopathy
  - Avoid heavy lifting
  - Avoid Valsalva-like maneuvers
  - Choose exercises that primarily involve the lower-extremity rather than upper-extremity muscle groups

and less stressful exercise regimens are recommended in these individuals. Strenuous exercise is contraindicated for patients with poor metabolic control and for those with significant diabetic complications (particularly active proliferative retinopathy, significant cardiovascular disease, and neuropathy).

BIBLIOGRAPHY

American Diabetes Association: Physical activity/exercise and diabetes (Position Statement). *Diabetes Care* 27 (Suppl. 1):S58–S62, 2004

DeFronzo R, Ferrannini E, Sato Y, Felig P, Wahren J: Synergistic interaction between exercise and insulin on peripheral glucose uptake. *J Clin Invest* 68:1468–1474, 1981

Fenicchia LM, Kanaley JA, Azevedo JL Jr, Miller CS, Weinstock RS, Carhart RL, Ploutz-Snyder LL: Influence of resistance exercise training on glucose control in women with type 2 diabetes. *Metabolism* 53:284–289, 2003

Kanaya AM, Narayan KM: Prevention of type 2 diabetes: data from recent trials. *Prim Care* 30:511–526, 2003

Maynard T: Physiological response to exercise in diabetes mellitus. *Diabetes Educ* 17:196–206, 1991

Petersen KF, Dufour S, Befroy D, Garcia R, Shulman GI: Impaired mitochondrial activity in the insulin-resistant offspring of patients with type 2 diabetes. *N Engl J Med* 350:664–671, 2004

Stewart KJ: Exercise training and the cardiovascular consequences of type 2 diabetes and hypertension. *JAMA* 288:1622–1631, 2002

Whelton SP, Chin A, Xin X, He J: Effect of aerobic exercise on blood pressure: a meta-analysis of randomized, controlled trials. *Ann Intern Med* 136:493–503, 2002

PHARMACOLOGIC INTERVENTION FOR GLYCEMIA

The last decade has brought major changes to the pharmacotherapy of type 2 diabetes. Four new classes of oral agents have been approved for use in the U.S., and new versions of sulfonylureas and insulin are available. Also, several factors now favor starting pharmacotherapy earlier, when glucose levels are only moderately elevated. First, the evidence that glycemic control is related to many complications of type 2 diabetes (as well as to those of type 1) is growing stronger. Second, the new definition of diabetes diagnosis, i.e., fasting plasma glucose (FPG) ≥126 mg/dl (≥7.0 mmol/l), has focused attention on less severely affected people who have previously not been identified or treated. Third, many of the new oral agents do not cause hypoglycemia when used alone, making early and more intensive treatment safer.

In general, pharmacologic intervention is considered only when optimal glucose control cannot be achieved with nutritional measures and regular exercise. However, because progressive β-cell dysfunction is related to persistent insulin resistance and persistent hyperinsulinemia, aggressive pharmacological therapy needs to be instituted quickly if the patient does not demonstrate a willingness to make lifestyle interventions or the ability to achieve glucose goals.

AVAILABLE AGENTS

The agents available for treating type 2 diabetes are listed in Table 3.7. They may be divided into two categories: those enhancing the effectiveness of insulin and those increasing the supply of insulin. Metformin, thiazolidinediones, and α-glucosidase inhibitors enhance the effectiveness of injected or endogenous insulin.

Table 3.7 Agents Available in the United States

Class	Generic Name	Brand Name
Enhancing the Effects of Insulin		
Biguanide	Metformin	Glucophage
Thiazolidinedione ("glitazone")	Rosiglitazone	Avandia
	Pioglitazone	Actos
α-Glucosidase inhibitor	Acarbose	Precose
	Miglitol	Glyset
Augmenting the Supply of Insulin		
Sulfonylurea	Tolbutamide	Orinase
	Chlorpropamide	Diabinese
	Tolazamide	Tolinase
	Glipizide	Glucotrol, Glucotrol XL
	Glyburide	DiaBeta, Micronase, Glynase
	Glimepiride	Amaryl
Nonsulfonylurea ("glinide")	Repaglinide	Prandin
	Nateglinide	Starlix

They have principal actions in the liver, adipose tissue and muscle, and the intestinal lumen, respectively, all assisting whatever insulin is available in regulating glucose levels. Sulfonylureas and the nonsulfonylurea secretagogues repaglinide and nateglinide as well as injected insulin increase the circulating levels of insulin. Sulfonylureas, repaglinide, and nateglinide increase the secretion of insulin into the portal circulation, whereas injected insulin supplements endogenously produced insulin levels in the systemic circulation. Because the mechanisms of action of all these classes of agents differ, except perhaps in the case of sulfonylureas and the nonsulfonylurea secretagogues, they may demonstrate complementary or additive effects in many cases.

Agents Enhancing the Effectiveness of Insulin

These agents are unlikely to cause hypoglycemia and can be used very early in the natural history of type 2 diabetes, so they are discussed first. Some features of these drugs are shown in Table 3.8.

Metformin. This agent belongs to the biguanide class of drugs. After administration, the highest concentrations of metformin are found in the gut and liver. It is not metabolized but rapidly cleared from plasma by the kidney. Because of rapid clearance, metformin is usually taken two or three times daily or in an extended-release formulation once or twice daily. Its mechanism of action is not completely understood, but its primary pharmacological effect is reducing elevated hepatic glucose production; it does not impair the ability of the patient to respond to fasting by increasing hepatic glucose production. It also may improve the response of muscle to insulin (especially at higher dosages) perhaps by reducing calorie intake or by alleviating "glucose toxicity" in muscles by lowering plasma glucose levels. Treatment with full dosage typically reduces A1C by 1–2%. When metformin is started, weight doesn't change or declines slightly, and lipid profiles and blood pressure may improve minimally.

The main risk of metformin treatment is lactic acidosis. However, experience suggests that fatal lactic acidosis associated with metformin is extremely rare, no more common than fatal hypoglycemia associated with sulfonylureas. To minimize this risk, metformin should not be given to patients with significant renal disease (serum creatinine >1.3 mg/dl for women, >1.5 mg/dl for men) or to those with serious hepatic or cardiovascular decompensation and should be used with caution in the elderly. Its main side effects are gastrointestinal, notably anorexia, nausea, or diarrhea. These side effects are frequent (10–30% of patients) at dosages >1,750 mg/day but may occur and persist at lower doses in ~5% of patients. In many patients, these side effects are transient and can be minimized by slow titration of the dose or alleviated by dose reduction when persistent.

Thiazolidinediones. The thiazolidinediones, more commonly referred to as glitazones, bind to PPAR-γ, a type of nuclear regulatory protein, altering the transcription of numerous genes believed to be important in fat and glucose metabolism. The metabolic effects of these agents develop gradually over several weeks and may take up to 3 months to reach full expression. The major site of action seems to be in adipose tissue, enhancing the expression of genes responsible for triglyceride storage. Glitazones may also initiate the development of new fat cells from stromal precursors, particularly in the subcutaneous compartment. The

Table 3.8 Characteristics of Therapies for Type 2 Diabetes

	Lifestyle	Insulins	Sulfonylureas	Metformin	α-Glucosidase Inhibitors	Rosiglitazone, Pioglitazone	Repaglinide, Nateglinide
Target tissue	Muscle/fat	β-cell supplement	β-cell	Liver	Gut	Fat, muscle, liver	β-cell
ΔA1C (monotherapy)	Variable	1 to >2%	1–2%	1–2%	0.5–1.0%	0.5–2.0%	1–2%
Fasting effect	Good	Excellent	Good	Good	Poor	Good	Good
Postprandial effect	Good	Excellent	Good	Good	Excellent	Good	Excellent
Hypoglycemia	Rare	Yes	Yes	Rare	No	Rare	Yes (R), Rare (N)
Dosing interval	Continuous	q.d. to continuous	q.d. to t.i.d.	b.i.d. or t.i.d.	b.i.d. to q.i.d.	q.d. or b.i.d.	b.i.d. to q.i.d.
ΔWeight (lb/yr)	+1	+3	+3	0 to –6	0 to –10	+1 to 13	+1
ΔInsulin	Variable	Increase	Increase	Modest decrease	Modest decrease	Decrease	Increase
ΔLDL cholesterol	Minimal decrease	Minimal decrease	None	Decrease	Minimal decrease	Increase (R), None (P)	None

Δ HDL cholesterol	Minimal increase	None	None	Increase	None	Increase	None
Δ Triglyceride	Minimal decrease	Decrease	None	Decrease	Minimal decrease	None (R), Decrease (P)	None
Common problem(s)	Recidivism, injury	Hypoglycemia, weight gain	Hypoglycemia, weight gain	Transient GI symptoms	Flatulence	Weight gain, edema, anemia	Hypoglycemia
Rare problem				Lactic acidosis		CHF	
Contraindications	None	None	Allergy	Renal failure, liver failure, CHF, age >80 yr	Intestinal disease	Hepatocellular disease, CHF	
Cost ($/mo)	0–200	15–45	5–40	40–80	25–50	75–200	30–60
Maximum effective dose		1–2 units/kg/day	½ max or double starting	1,000 mg b.i.d.	50 t.i.d. acarbose, 25 t.i.d. miglitol	Max dose on package insert	2 mg t.i.d.

GI, gastrointestinal; CHF, congestive heart failure.

increase in the ability to store triglyceride results in a reduction in serum free fatty acid concentrations and a net shift of fat from other tissues such as muscle, liver, and β-cells, resulting in an improvement in insulin action and insulin secretion. The glitazones can also alter the expression of a number of "adipokines," which also may result in improvement in insulin action (see Chapter 2, Pathogenesis).

Troglitazone was the first thiazolidinedione approved for clinical use in the U.S.; however, it was withdrawn from the market as a result of rare cases of severe hepatotoxicity. The remaining agents, rosiglitazone and pioglitazone, appear not to have hepatotoxicity. Nevertheless, it is suggested that these agents not be used in patients with active liver disease or in patients with transaminases elevated >2.5-fold over the upper limits of normal and that intermittent liver function test monitoring be performed.

The glitazones are associated with reductions of A1C on the order of 1–2%, reducing both fasting and postprandial glucose substantially. Due to their insulin-sensitizing nature, they are associated with a reduction in glucose with either no change or a reduction in insulin levels. These agents also have effects on β-cell function and are associated with a normalization of the proinsulin-to-insulin ratio and improved β-cell secretory dynamics and reactivity. Treatment with glitazones may also slow the rate of decline of β-cell function observed in patients treated with a sulfonylurea or metformin. These may be important effects and suggest that these agents may provide more durable responses with less secondary failure than other antidiabetic treatments.

Fluid retention and weight gain have been the main adverse events in human trials of glitazones. The weight gain is least when the glitazones are used in combination with diet and exercise or with metformin (generally a few pounds over the first year versus placebo) and greater when these agents are used in combination with insulin or sulfonylurea (average weight gain on the order of 5–10 lb over the first year). The fluid retention most commonly results in edema. Cases of congestive heart failure (CHF) have been precipitated by glitazone treatment. The patients presenting with CHF often have diastolic dysfunction as the underlying cardiac performance problem, and many such patients are asymptomatic. There is no evidence in humans that there is an untoward effect of glitazones on cardiac performance. It is recommended that patients on insulin, with peripheral edema, or who have a history of cardiac disease be started on the lowest dose of glitazone and the dose titrated slowly, with monitoring of therapeutic response and potential side effects. Patients should be educated regarding the possibility of fluid retention presenting as edema, dyspnea, or fatigue and should be counseled to return for evaluation should these problems develop. Diuretics seem to work to minimize symptomatology. There is anecdotal evidence that the risk of fluid retention is higher in patients treated with nonsteroidal anti-inflammatory drugs and calcium-channel blockers and perhaps less in those treated with angiotensin-converting enzyme (ACE) inhibitors, angiotensin receptor blockers (ARBs), or diuretics, but this has not been systematically studied in clinical trials. Glitazones are contraindicated in patients with class III or class IV heart failure because of these concerns and the lack of studies to evaluate their safety and efficacy in those populations.

Glitazones also seem to have favorable effects on circulating lipids. Rosiglitazone is associated with an elevation in serum HDL cholesterol and LDL cholesterol particle size with a moderate increase in LDL cholesterol levels. Pioglitazone is associated with improvements in serum HDL cholesterol, triglycerides, and LDL cholesterol particle size with no change in LDL cholesterol levels versus placebo. Both agents have been demonstrated to have moderate-to-substantial effects on numerous inflammatory and cellular markers associated with excess cardiovascular risk. Although there are no studies that directly demonstrate a reduction in cardiovascular events, this class of drugs does demonstrate substantial promise to provide long-term cardiovascular benefits.

α-Glucosidase inhibitors. Acarbose and miglitol are α-glucosidase inhibitors, which work in the intestinal lumen, where they competitively inhibit enzymes that hydrolyze polysaccharides into simple sugars. Their main effect is on starches, but cleavage of the disaccharide sucrose to glucose and fructose is also reduced. Cleavage of lactose is unaffected. The result of this action is to delay absorption of dietary carbohydrates until they have passed to the mid or distal small bowel, resulting in reduced postprandial peaks of plasma glucose. They have little effect on fasting glucose. To achieve this effect, the tablets must be taken at the beginning of meals. In general, the resulting overall glycemic reduction is modest, with A1C changes of 0.5–1.0%. Acarbose is largely not absorbed from the intestine, whereas miglitol is. The major adverse effects are flatulence, abdominal distress or distension, and diarrhea. These result from excessive blockade of carbohydrate absorption in the small bowel, leading to fermentation and gas production in the colon. They are minimized by low initial dosage with gradual titration upward. Intestinal distension or diarrhea may be harmful in the presence of inflammatory bowel disease or other major intestinal disorders.

Agents Augmenting the Supply of Insulin

Sulfonylureas and nonsulfonylurea insulin secretagogues. These agents are only effective in the presence of endogenous insulin production. They exert their antidiabetic effects through their interaction with a cell surface protein termed the sulfonylurea receptor (SUR), which regulates the activity of potassium channels. Binding of sulfonylureas and nonsulfonylureas results in closure of potassium channels and depolarization of the membrane, opening calcium channels and stimulating insulin release. In the β-cell, binding of insulin secretagogues increases insulin secretion in a relatively glucose-independent fashion, resulting in a reduction of fasting glucose as well as a proportional reduction of the postprandial rise of glucose. The net effect is generally a 1–2% reduction in A1C, the exception being nateglinide, which is associated with a 0.5–1.0% reduction as a result of its short half-life and residence time on the sulfonylurea receptor.

The main complication of sulfonylurea treatment is hypoglycemia. Elderly patients are more susceptible, especially when they have declining renal function or tend to skip meals. The risk of hypoglycemia seems to be related to both the pharmacologic half-life and the details of the interaction of the drug with the sulfonylurea receptor. Glyburide seems to be associated with a higher risk of hypoglycemia than glimepiride, repaglinide, nateglinide, or sustained-release formulations of glipizide. In patients with modest hyperglycemia, particularly when treated with insulin sensitizers, starting with the lowest possible dose is an important safety consideration.

Other side effects are uncommon, but the leading ones are gastrointestinal symptoms, such as nausea and vomiting; and skin reactions, including rashes, purpura, and pruritis. Rare side effects include hematologic reactions (leukopenia, thrombocytopenia, or hemolytic anemia) and cholestasis (with or without jaundice). Modest weight gain may occur when treatment is started.

Some features of sulfonylureas available in the U.S. are shown in Table 3.9. The first-generation sulfonylureas (tolbutamide, tolazamide, and chlorpropamide) bind significantly to plasma proteins and have high milligram dosage requirements. Because of the protein binding, they can displace or be displaced by other agents, such as salicylates or warfarin, leading to drug interactions. Tolbutamide is rapidly cleared by the liver and must be taken two or three times daily. Chlorpropamide is slowly cleared by the kidney and accumulates, particularly when renal function declines, and as a result may cause serious hypoglycemia. Chlorpropamide also may cause an antabuse-like intolerance to alcohol or potentiate antidiuretic hormone action leading to water intoxication. Because of these limitations, the first-generation agents are not commonly used.

The second-generation sulfonylureas (glyburide, glipizide, and glimepiride) are largely free of interactions with other drugs and have lower total dosage requirements. They are metabolized mainly by the liver and cleared renally, except glimepiride, which is excreted by both renal and hepatic mechanisms. Glyburide

Table 3.9 Characteristics of Sulfonylureas

Generic Name	Brand Name	Approved Daily Dosage Range (mg)	Near Maximum Effective Dosage (mg)	Duration of Action (h)	Clearance
Tolbutamide	Orinase	500–3,000	1,000 t.i.d.	6–12	Hepatic
Chlorpropamide	Diabinese	100–500	500 q.d.	>48	Renal
Tolazamide	Tolinase	100–1,000	500 b.i.d.	12–24	Hepatic, renal
Glipizide	Glucotrol	2.5–40	10 b.i.d.	12–18	Hepatic
	Glucotrol XL (extended release)	2.5–20	10 q.d.	24	Hepatic
Glyburide	DiaBeta	1.25–20	5 b.i.d.	12–24	Hepatic
	Micronase	1.25–2	5 b.i.d.	12–24	Hepatic, renal
	Glynase	0.75–12	3 b.i.d.	12–24	Hepatic, renal
Glimepiride	Amaryl	1–8	4 q.d.	24	Hepatic or renal
Repaglinide	Prandin	1–16	4 t.i.d.	2–6	Hepatic
Nateglinide	Starlix	60–360	120 t.i.d.	2–4	Hepatic, renal

has an active metabolite that must be excreted by the kidney. Thus, in the setting of renal insufficiency, glyburide is associated with greater concern and glimepiride with fewer issues from a drug metabolism perspective. Both glyburide and glipizide require twice-daily doses to produce 24-h coverage, although glipizide is available in an extended-release formulation that is fully effective given once a day.

The newest insulin secretagogues are nonsulfonylurea agents (the "glinides"). Their action is mediated through the SUR, and they hold some structural homology to the sulfonylureas but do not contain the actual sulfonylurea moiety. Both repaglinide and nateglinide are rapidly absorbed after oral administration and rapidly cleared by hepatic metabolism. This rapid time course of action calls for two or three doses daily with meals. Repaglinide is able to reduce fasting levels of glucose despite its short half-life because of prolonged residence on the SUR complex and thus can reduce A1C equivalent to sulfonylureas. Nateglinide, on the other hand, has a short residence time and does not substantially reduce fasting glucose. As a result, it is the secretagogue that most specifically lowers postprandial glucose with a minimal risk of hypoglycemia. However, because of its lack of effect on fasting glucose, its efficacy in lowering A1C is modest.

Whether insulin secretagogues that work through the SUR have significant effects beyond the β-cell has been debated. After chronic sulfonylurea treatment, the peripheral tissues can become more sensitive to insulin, but this seems largely due to waning of the adverse effects of hyperglycemia (glucotoxicity). Sulfonylureas bind to potassium channels in various tissues, including vascular tissue, and may reduce vasodilation. Whether this effect is clinically important is unknown. There have been studies suggesting the possibility that sulfonylureas could adversely affect cardiac rhythm in the setting of ischemia that may result in dysrhythmias. This seems to be less of a concern with glimepiride, sustained-release preparations of glipizide, and the nonsulfonylurea secretagogues repaglinide and nateglinide than with glyburide.

Insulin

Although insulin has been used therapeutically for >70 years, some aspects of its use are new. Insulins extracted from the pancreases of cattle and pigs are no longer generally available. They have largely been replaced by insulin that is synthesized by genetically altered bacteria or yeast and structurally identical to human insulin. The familiar extended-action preparations (NPH, lente, and ultralente) are still available (Table 3.10), but their onset and duration of action are shorter when made from human rather than animal insulin. This difference is less apparent in treatment of type 2 diabetes than with type 1 diabetes, because absorption of insulin after subcutaneous injection is generally slower in type 2 patients, and response is blunted by insulin resistance.

There are now five structurally modified variants of human insulin, so-called insulin analogs approved by the Food and Drug Administration. Three are rapid-acting insulin analogs. Insulins lispro, aspart, and glulisine (which has received FDA approval but is not yet being marketed) each involve a different structural modification that disrupts the "tail structure" of the insulin molecule. As a result, these forms of insulin do not exhibit as great a tendency to form dimers and hexamers at high concentration. The net effect is that they are more rapidly absorbed

Table 3.10 Characteristics of Human Insulins and Analogs

Preparation	Trade Name	Timing of Action		
		Onset	Peak	Duration
Short-acting				
Lispro, aspart, glulisine	Humalog, Novolog, Apidra	5 min	0.5–1 h	3 h
Regular	Humulin R, Novolin R	30 min	2–5 h	5–8 h
Intermediate-acting				
NPH	Humulin N, Novolin N	1–2 h	6–10 h	16–24+ h
Lente	Humulin L, Novolin L	1–2 h	8–12 h	18–24+ h
Long-acting				
Glargine	Lantus	~2 h	None	~24 h
Ultralente	Humulin U	4–6 h	10–18 h	16–24+ h
Detemir	Levemir	1–2 h	2–12 h	16–24+ h
Mixtures				
70/30, 50/50, 75/25	Various	30 min	7–12 h	16–24+ h

This table summarizes the typical time course of various insulin preparations based on contributors' clinical expertise. Values are highly variable among individuals. Even in an individual, values vary depending on the site and depth of injection, skin temperature, and exercise.

after subcutaneous injection compared to regular insulin, starting to work in 5–15 min and peaking in 30–60 min with an effective duration of action of 3–6 h. Whereas regular human insulin should ideally be administered ≥30 min before meals, these analogs should be administered just before meals or even after meals when the amount of carbohydrate is not known before eating. In general, these rapid-acting insulin analogs are associated with a somewhat lower risk of hypoglycemia, with occasional studies demonstrating greater improvements in A1C than with regular insulin.

There are two long-acting insulin analogs. Glargine insulin has been modified to form a precipitate at neutral pH. It is supplied as a clear, colorless solution at acidic pH and on subcutaneous injection precipitates with slow dissolution, producing essentially peakless action over ~24 h. Studies have demonstrated that in patients not reaching optimal glycemic control with oral agents, administration of glargine once nightly is associated with identical overall control assessed by A1C compared to NPH insulin with a lower risk of hypoglycemia, particularly during the night. Insulin detemir has an approvable letter from the FDA but is not yet marketed. Its structure is modified by acylation so that the resulting structure is bound to fatty acid–binding sites in tissues and on albumin. In contrast to glargine, insulin detemir is absorbed rapidly but displays prolonged action as a result of it circulating largely in a bound form while activity is only associated with the free fraction that can cross the endothelium to bind to tissue insulin receptors. Unlike glargine, detemir can be mixed with rapid-acting insulin.

Premixed combinations of insulins are available and widely used. Those sold in the U.S. are 70/30 (70% NPH and 30% regular) and 50/50 (50% NPH and

50% regular) insulins as well as mixtures of NPH and analogs. These fixed combinations have serious limitations for patients with type 1 diabetes, who need to modify insulin doses per insulin-to-carbohydrate ratios and carbohydrate intake frequently. In contrast, many patients with type 2 diabetes have substantial endogenous insulin and can use premixed insulin both conveniently, with less time spent preparing the dose, and effectively, with optimal glycemic results.

Insulin has essentially unlimited power to reduce plasma glucose. It reduces blood glucose level by suppressing hepatic glucose production and by increasing glucose uptake by insulin-sensitive tissues, notably muscle and adipose tissue. As with sulfonylureas, the improved glycemic control achieved with insulin therapy generally increases the responsiveness of tissues to insulin. The main practical limitation in achieving treatment objectives with insulin is the risk of hypoglycemia. Also, patients with type 2 diabetes, who are typically already obese, usually gain weight when insulin treatment is started. Other side effects include immediate skin reactions at injection sites (itching, redness, and swelling) or persistent lumps or swelling at these sites that may represent delayed hypersensitivity reactions. These allergy-related problems are less common with current insulin preparations than with previous ones and may be less common in people with type 2 diabetes than in those with type 1 diabetes.

SELECTING AN AGENT TO BEGIN TREATMENT

With more agents to choose from, pharmacotherapy of type 2 diabetes has become both more effective and more complex over the last decade. Different agents have different clinical effects (Table 3.8). The first treatment decision is required when a patient is found, despite the best possible effort with lifestyle modification, to have an A1C >7% or fasting glucose levels >108 mg/dl (>6.0 mmol/l). The UKPDS demonstrated that the groups with 10-year median A1C values of ~7% were associated with better outcomes than those with median A1C values of 8%. The treatment protocol in the UKPDS held that if a patient had a fasting glucose >108 mg/dl (>6.0 mmol/l), they were eligible for randomization. Those patients randomized to continue on lifestyle intervention had poorer outcomes than those randomized to medications. Thus, the evidence would suggest that drug therapy is indicated if fasting glucose cannot be controlled to levels <108 mg/dl despite best lifestyle efforts for 3 months. There are no similar trials that provide similar cut points for postprandial glucose levels associated with improved outcomes.

Fasting Plasma Glucose <130 mg/dl (<7.2 mmol/l)

Patients with relatively modest elevations of FPG despite their best efforts at lifestyle changes should probably be preferentially treated with agents not associated with hypoglycemia risk. Metformin arguably is the best studied agent for the treatment of diabetes. As discussed above, it is not associated with weight gain and was associated with reduced cardiovascular events among overweight patients randomized in the UKPDS. The glitazone agents are generally better tolerated, although more expensive and less well studied. They show tremendous promise as agents that may be associated with a lower rate of secondary failure due to progression of β-cell dysfunction as well as a reduction in cardiovascular disease rate;

however, there is no proof in this regard. The α-glucosidase inhibitors are not associated with hypoglycemia or weight gain but have not been widely used in most countries in part because of cultural stigma regarding the most common adverse effect—flatulence. That said, there is substantial reason to believe that these agents are beneficial and should be considered. Among the insulin secretagogues, nateglinide has the lowest potential for severe hypoglycemia and would be a reasonable choice, particularly in patients with near-normal fasting glucose. Extended-release glipizide or glimepiride or another sulfonylurea could be tried at the lowest possible dose, although many patients will have symptomatic hypoglycemia at least intermittently. Finally, insulin therapy is not out of the question at this level of glycemic control, although it would rarely be the leading choice of many patients or providers.

In each case, the adverse effects and contraindications should be carefully reviewed. The dosage should be started low and titrated upward slowly. The starting dose of metformin is 500 mg one or two times daily with breakfast and/or the evening meal. After 1–2 weeks, the dose may be increased sequentially until unacceptable adverse effects arise or the patient is taking an adequate or the maximally tolerated dose of 1,000 mg b.i.d. It is generally better tolerated when taken with a meal. The glitazones should be started at the lowest dose with follow-up generally in 4–12 weeks. It will generally take 2–4 weeks to see much of a response in self-monitored blood glucose and 3–6 months to see the full A1C benefit. With the α-glucosidase inhibitors, a program analogous to that described with metformin should be initiated starting with the smallest available tablet once daily with the first bite of the largest meal. Every 2–4 weeks, an additional tablet can be added until the drug is taken at each main meal. Subsequently, the dose of the tablet can be increased, but similar to the sulfonylureas, there is rarely a substantial response with regard to efficacy as the highest doses are approached, whereas the adverse effects generally worsen proportionately with the dose; generally, 50 mg t.i.d. will provide a maximal effect.

Fasting Plasma Glucose >130 mg/dl (>7.2 mmol/l)

In this situation, the aforementioned options will also apply, although in general, the ability of the more postprandially targeted oral approaches (α-glucosidase inhibitors and glinides) will often not produce adequate overall control. Sulfonylureas are much less likely to be associated with substantial problems with frequent or severe hypoglycemia, particularly if the patient starts with a low dose. The dose of a sulfonylurea can be increased with just a few days of experience because they work very quickly at maximal effect. Maximal clinical effectiveness is usually reached at half the maximal labeled dose of sulfonylurea.

Consideration can also be given to initiating two agents in this setting, particularly if A1C is >9% or FPG is >200 mg/dl, because a single agent will not usually produce an adequate reduction in glucose. In general, a combination of agents that improves insulin action (metformin, glitazones, or α-glucosidase inhibitors) with a secretagogue will be more potent in reducing A1C than a combination without a secretagogue. That said, the combination of metformin with a glitazone is quite compelling in that there should be very low risk of hypoglycemia or weight gain as well as the potential of improved cardiovascular outcomes. There are several branded combinations of oral antidiabetic agents. They provide substantial convenience and perhaps the potential for better adherence but allow less flexibility in dosing and dose adjustment and, in most circumstances, are more expensive.

Insulin may also be used for initial treatment of type 2 diabetes, although most patients prefer to use oral treatments first. Strong consideration for initial therapy with insulin should be considered in patients with A1Cs substantially >10% or with FPG levels ≥300 mg/dl (≥16.7 mmol/l). Initiation of insulin treatment will be described later in this chapter.

PRIMARY AND SECONDARY FAILURE OF TREATMENTS

In some cases, a treatment may fail when first tried. This has been called primary failure, and in some cases it indicates incorrect selection of the treatment. For example, none of the oral agents will work well in a patient with type 1 diabetes. It is worth remembering that current estimates suggest that up to 10% of adult-onset diabetes is in fact a slowly evolving form of type 1 diabetes. Failure is also common when FPG is well over 300 mg/dl (>16.7 mmol/l) and A1C >10% when an oral agent is started; thus, there is the recommendation to start therapy with insulin with the notion that oral agents can be added later and an effort made to discontinue insulin if desired by both the patient and provider.

Even if effective from the beginning, any therapy for type 2 diabetes becomes less effective over time. This also applies to lifestyle changes and insulin. Secondary failure of treatments is related to progression of the underlying abnormalities of β-cell function and insulin action. The UKPDS showed that, with continuous treatment, A1C increases at a rate averaging 0.2%/year or 1% over 5 years. Thus, a treatment successfully reducing A1C from 7.5 to 6.5% is likely to show secondary failure, defined as a return to the initial level of control, within 5 years. Substituting another oral agent for the one no longer fully effective is rarely helpful in this situation. As mentioned, this rate of failure seems to be lower in 1- and 2-year studies with glitazones than with sulfonylurea and metformin.

It seems evident that many patients could progress to treatment with up to four classes of oral antidiabetic agents. In fact, there is no substantial experience with four-drug therapy. There are several studies that address the combination of metformin, a glitazone, and a secretagogue with substantial efficacy, the final oral agent added lowering A1C by ~1%. However, patients treated with three-drug regimens often do not achieve A1C <7%. Thus, the alternative of proceeding directly to insulin therapy or using a combination of insulin and oral agents should be considered. As with antihypertensive drugs, many patients require multiple oral agents to attain adequate glycemic control. Numerous studies using two hyperglycemic agents have shown significant efficacy when one agent fails. Importantly, studies have also shown that the second agent should be added instead of exchanging one agent for another. Particularly effective is a sulfonylurea with either metformin or a glitazone.

STARTING INSULIN THERAPY

Insulin is capable of restoring glycemia to near normal in most patients with type 2 diabetes. Although this therapy may result in elevated insulin levels, there is little direct evidence that insulin itself leads to further complications, especially cardiovascular disease. In fact, substantial evidence supports insulin therapy in the setting of hyperglycemia as associated with improved outcomes, including a long-term study in ambulatory patients with type 1 or type 2 diabetes, as well as in the setting of acute myocardial infarction and intensive care management. Therefore, the focus should be on glucose control rather than on the theoretical deleterious effects of hyperinsulinemia. In fact, there are also physicians who have a clear-cut preference for insulin to oral hypoglycemic agents as the primary pharmacologic intervention, after diet and exercise alone are no longer successful. Insulin is particularly appropriate as primary therapy for patients with rapid uncontrolled weight loss unexplained by diet who also have severe hyperglycemia, especially when accompanied by ketonemia or ketonuria. Such patients may be severely insulin deficient and, in fact, have late-onset type 1 diabetes rather than type 2 diabetes.

Other indications for the use of insulin include

- periods of acute injury, stress, infection, surgery, or glucocorticoid treatment
- pregnancy
- renal or hepatic disease or allergies that preclude use of oral therapies
- primary or secondary failure of oral agents

Note that any metabolic state or drug that increases the requirement for insulin or interferes with insulin secretion may require temporary insulin therapy. Management with insulin during pregnancy or surgery is discussed in Chapter 4, Special Therapeutic Situations. Insulin therapy should be used with particular care in poorly adherent patients who are unwilling or unable to perform SMBG or patients for whom hypoglycemia is a serious risk, such as those with cerebrovascular disease or unstable angina.

Because the tissues of patients with type 2 diabetes are usually less responsive to insulin, large doses of insulin may be necessary. This is particularly true for severely obese patients with type 2 diabetes, who may require 100–200 units/day or more. More than one daily injection is usually required. Note that an approach in which insulin injections are added as required by overall control is generally better accepted by most patients than beginning with two or more injections daily. Starting insulin is a milestone in a person's experience living with diabetes. It requires education and emotional support and more careful monitoring of glucose because of the possibility of hypoglycemia. The tactics for starting insulin may vary somewhat, depending on whether oral agents are already being used.

Insulin Without Oral Agents

When starting insulin in patients not taking oral agents, a single injection of intermediate- or long-acting insulin may be given either before breakfast or at bedtime. Patients with predominantly daytime hyperglycemia, who begin the day with a fasting glucose level close to target that rises with each meal, are likely to respond better to a morning injection, and those with substantial fasting hyperglycemia may be candidates for a bedtime injection. In randomized trials, the evening insulin approach in the setting of type 2 diabetes has generally been associated with improved control and less weight gain.

For the average overweight uncontrolled patient, a conservative starting dose of 10 units at bedtime is unlikely to cause hypoglycemia yet will improve glycemia somewhat while the patient is learning to handle and inject insulin. Glucose monitoring by SMBG should be done at least every morning, with occasional monitoring at other times of the day to determine whether glucose levels rise during the day or there is unrecognized hypoglycemia. A recent study demonstrated that a simple algorithm to drive once-weekly titration of bedtime NPH or glargine works well with professional supervision. In the Treat-to-Target Trial, if no fasting glucose <72 mg/dl (<4 mmol/l), no severe hypoglycemia, and no glucose <56 mg/dl (<3.1 mmol/l) was documented in the prior week, the average of the previous 2 days' fasting glucose levels was used to drive the increase. If the average fasting glucose was >180 mg/dl (>10 mmol/l), the bedtime dose was increased by 8 units/day. If the average was 140–180 mg/dl (7.8–10.0 mmol/l), the dose was increased by 6 units. If the average was 120–140 mg/dl (6.7–7.8 mmol/l), the dose was increased by 4 units, and if it was 100–120 mg/dl (5.6–6.7 mmol/l), the dose was increased 2 units. An alternative approach is to ask patients to increase their dose of insulin by 1 unit/day whenever fasting glucose is >100 mg/dl and decrease it by 2–4 units for fasting glucose <80 mg/dl. Table 3.11 provides some additional considerations for monitoring if bedtime insulin is not the initial regimen prescribed.

Some patients will have excellent responses with a single injection and may maintain target levels of control this way for some time. In other cases, two daily injections will be required for best results. Generally, a mixture of intermediate- and rapid- or short-acting insulins should be given before breakfast and before the evening meal. The ratio of the morning to evening doses needed varies among patients. Some need up to two-thirds of the total in the morning, others need two-thirds in the evening, and many need approximately equal amounts at each injection.

Table 3.11 Insulin Regimen and Timing of Self-Monitoring of Blood Glucose

Insulin	Time Injected	Period of Greatest Activity	Blood Check Reflecting Insulin Action
Rapid- or Short-acting	Before a meal	Between that meal and the next meal or bed-time	Just before the next meal; occasionally 1–2 h after injection
Intermediate-acting	Before breakfast	Between lunch and evening meal	Before lunch and supper
	Before evening meal	Between midnight and breakfast	Before bedtime, midsleep, and breakfast
Long-acting	At bedtime	Between 4 a.m. and breakfast	Before breakfast
	Before breakfast or bedtime	Mostly overnight, because short-acting insulin overrides its effect during the day	Before breakfast

The same is true of the ratio of intermediate- to rapid- or short-acting insulin at each dose. Some patients do very well with a 2-to-1 ratio; others do better with a 1-to-1 ratio. A simple and reasonable way to begin two-injection treatment is with 10 units premixed 70/30 insulin (70% NPH, 30% regular) or 75/25 (75% NPL, 25% lispro) twice daily. Both the dosage and distribution should be modified as indicated by the SMBG results. Relatively nonobese patients may achieve good glucose control with no more than 20–40 units daily. Obese patients will need more, often 100–200 units daily. Many patients will need to mix intermediate- and rapid- or short-acting insulins from separate vials to vary the ratio for optimal results.

The alternative approach is to use a multiple daily injection (MDI) regimen analogous to the techniques commonly used to treat type 1 diabetes. This method provides the greatest flexibility on the part of the patient and with the advent of insulin pens, is convenient even with the most active lifestyles. MDI is generally required in two circumstances: for hypoglycemia with activity or delayed meals and for rising glucose levels during the day, despite achieving adequate control of fasting glucose. In transitioning from one injection to two or more, there is one very important safety consideration: If the patient's fasting glucose is well controlled, care should be taken as the second or subsequent injection is added to avoid the development of nocturnal or morning hypoglycemia. In this circumstance, it is prudent to reduce the long-acting insulin dose by 10–25% as the rapid-acting insulin is added. In addition, patients should be reminded of the relationship between carbohydrate intake and meal-related insulin requirements. The insulin regimen that provides for excellent glycemic control after a breakfast of cereal and juice will certainly result in hypoglycemia after bacon and eggs. Two techniques for dealing with this relationship include setting a fixed intake of carbohydrate at each main meal or using the technique of carbohydrate counting. In the latter, patients are instructed to count either servings or grams of carbohydrate in their meals and are provided with a dose of insulin to administer per serving or gram of carbohydrate. In general, starting at 1 unit insulin per carbohydrate serving or 1 unit per 15 grams of carbohydrate is reasonable. Most patients with type 2 diabetes will require 2–5 units per 15-gram serving of carbohydrate. There are many available carbohydrate counting guides to assist in this process (visit http://store. diabetes.org for tools and books published by the American Diabetes Association). Patients generally rapidly adapt to this technique because the number of food choices that most patients consume over a period of weeks are remarkably limited, and mastery of the carbohydrate content of these commonly eaten foods develops quickly. In patients with type 2 diabetes, injections with each meal may not be needed. For example, a patient may do well on a regimen of long-acting insulin at bedtime with rapid-acting insulin at breakfast in the setting of a carbohydrate-rich breakfast, a lunch modest in carbohydrate content, and physical activity during the day. Some patients will only require rapid-acting insulin with dinner. The advantages of this technique are numerous because it provides great flexibility and also highlights the relationship of dietary intake with glycemic control.

It is worth mentioning that continuous insulin infusion (insulin pump therapy) is an alternative to insulin injection in the setting of type 2 diabetes. Studies to date have not demonstrated the superiority of insulin pump therapy, particularly in type 2 diabetes. However, for patients whose dietary habit is to graze during the day and who have difficulty adhering to a routine of administering insulin with each snack, insulin pump therapy can be remarkably more effective as it allows patients to administer insulin an unlimited number of times during the day as they eat quickly and conveniently.

Insulin After Failure of Oral Agents

The task of starting insulin is slightly different when oral agents have been used and secondary failure has ensued. There are two options. The traditional option is to stop oral agents and begin insulin alone. However, after secondary failure of oral agents, insulin must be used more aggressively than when it is the initial treatment. The reason for this is that by the time secondary failure of oral agents has occurred, the underlying defects of insulin secretion and action have progressed, and withdrawing oral agents may lead to rapid loss of glycemic control. Some believe that a single injection of insulin is unlikely to be effective, and two injections should be started immediately, at a dosage of 10–15 units twice daily. On the other hand, the Treat-to-Target Trial demonstrated that patients with secondary failure on one or two oral agents were able to achieve A1C <7% more than 50% of the time with one injection of bedtime NPH or glargine. However, note that although these patients' glucose levels throughout the course of the day were not normal, their average glucose levels over months were sufficiently low to reach the A1C goal. The dosage should be increased at frequent intervals, such as every 2–3 days, guided by the results of SMBG.

The second option is to add insulin to the prior oral regimen; in general, this is simpler and arguably more effective. Again, available clinical trial data suggest that once-daily glargine or NPH at bedtime or, in obese patients, 70/30 insulin before the evening meal is more effective than alternative approaches. The rationale is that supplementing with overnight insulin will control fasting hyperglycemia, while continuing the oral agents will prevent worsening of glycemic control during the time that the insulin dosage is titrated upward.

LONG-TERM COMBINATIONS OF ORAL AGENTS WITH INSULIN

By the time oral agents have failed, β-cell function has usually declined enough that sulfonylureas provide little benefit and can be stopped. Note that a few patients are able to maintain glycemic control better through the day on regimens involving morning sulfonylureas versus a single injection of insulin at night. Studies have demonstrated that the degree of glucose lowering is on average greater when insulin is added to a glitazone than when insulin is used alone. The combination of insulin and metformin is associated with less weight gain than when insulin is used alone. Certainly, the continued use of oral agents can reduce the total insulin dosage, sometimes preventing the need to use more than a single 100-unit syringeful at a given time of day. For these reasons, continuing agents that enhance insulin action may be given serious consideration.

The effect of combining metformin or a glitazone with or without a sulfonylurea with insulin is best seen when one of these agents is either added to or withdrawn from previously established insulin treatment. There are substantial numbers of patients who are treated with insulin alone who have never received metformin or a glitazone. In such patients, perhaps one-third to one-half can be withdrawn from insulin and placed on combined oral agent therapy by reducing the dose of insulin sequentially by 10–25% as oral agents are titrated in while glucose levels remain in the target range.

ADJUSTING INSULIN DOSAGE IN LONG-TERM TYPE 2 DIABETES

By 15–20 years after the onset of type 2 diabetes, many patients have markedly reduced endogenous insulin secretion. At this time, glycemic variability increases and reliance on injected insulin becomes greater. Therefore, treatment of these patients becomes more like that of type 1 diabetes than it was earlier in the course of their type 2 diabetes. Both the patient and physician must be aware of the time course of action of the various kinds of insulin and the times at which hypoglycemia is most likely to occur. Blood glucose levels must be monitored at home regularly by the patient or a responsible helper, and adjustments of meal pattern and/or insulin made when necessary.

Table 3.11 shows the times at which different kinds of injected insulin are most active in reducing glucose levels when given at various times of day. Rapid- or short-acting insulin is given before meals and is active during the interval up to 3–4 h after the meal (in the case of the rapid-acting analogs) and ≥6 h after the meal (in the case of regular insulin). Intermediate-acting insulin has peak activity 6–12 h after injection. Because intermediate-acting insulin is commonly given before breakfast, before the evening meal, or at bedtime, it may cause hypoglycemia in the late afternoon, from midnight to 4 a.m., or just before breakfast.

Four different insulin regimens are shown in Table 3.12. Regimen 1 is the two-injection regimen using both intermediate-acting and rapid- or short-acting insulin described previously. It is effective for many patients with type 2 diabetes as long as they retain significant endogenous insulin secretion. The dosages used

Table 3.12 Sample Insulin Regimens for Achieving Glycemic Control

	Before Breakfast	Before Lunch	Before Evening Meal	Bedtime
1	Intermediate- + rapid- or short-acting		Intermediate- + rapid- or short-acting	
2	Intermediate- + rapid- or short-acting		Rapid- or short-acting	Intermediate-acting
3	Intermediate- + rapid- or short-acting	Rapid- or short-acting	Rapid- or short-acting	Intermediate-acting
4	Rapid- or short-acting	Rapid- or short-acting	Rapid- or short-acting	Long-acting

at each injection can be adjusted on the basis of SMBG results. Disproportionately high values before lunch suggest inadequate rapid- or short-acting insulin in the morning injection, and high values at bedtime suggest that the rapid- or short-acting insulin given before the evening meal is insufficient. Similarly, high glucose levels before the evening meal or breakfast suggest the need to increase the morning or evening intermediate-acting dose, respectively. Low glucose values suggest excessive dosage of the insulins responsible for coverage at each of these times of day. When adjustments of individual components of the insulin regimen are necessary, premixed insulins are less effective, and better results will be obtained if the patient mixes the insulins for each injection.

Regimen 2 differs from regimen 1 in that the intermediate-acting insulin has been moved from the evening meal to bedtime. The advantage of this change is to reduce the chance of hypoglycemia between midnight and 4 a.m. by shifting the peak effect of the dose closer to breakfast. This change is necessary mostly for active, less obese patients who absorb insulin rapidly and may develop nocturnal hypoglycemia on the two-injection regimen.

Regimens 3 and 4 are full multiple daily injection regimens that may be desirable for patients who tend to have widely variable SMBG readings in the late afternoon when using regimen 2. Moving part of the rapid- or short-acting dose given at breakfast to lunchtime generally smooths afternoon control. Regimen 4 offers the greatest flexibility with eating and exercise patterns and can be highly individualized, provided the patient is willing to match insulin dose to carbohydrate intake and perform SMBG. For example, some older people awaken late and eat just two meals, the first (and sometimes main) meal close to midday and a second meal in the evening. In this case, the first insulin injection may best be given before the midday meal and the second before the evening meal.

BIBLIOGRAPHY

American Diabetes Association: Insulin administration (Position Statement). *Diabetes Care* 27 (Suppl. 1):S106–S109, 2004

DeFronzo RA, Goodman AM, the Multicenter Metformin Study Group: Efficacy of metformin in patients with non-insulin-dependent diabetes mellitus. *N Engl J Med* 333:541–549, 1995

Edelman SV: The role of the thiazolidinediones in the practical management of patients with type 2 diabetes and cardiovascular risk factors. *Rev Cardiovasc Med* 4 (Suppl. 6):S29–S37, 2003

Edelman SV, Henry RR: Intensive insulin therapy for patients with type II diabetes. In *Diabetes Mellitus: A Fundamental and Clinical Text.* LeRoith D, Taylor SI, Olefsky JM, Eds. Philadelphia, Lippincott-Raven, 1996, p. 647–660

Garber AJ, Duncan TG, Goodman AM, Mills DJ, Rohlf JL: Efficacy of metformin in type 2 diabetes: results of a double-blind, placebo-controlled, dose-response trial. *Am J Med* 103:491–497, 1997

Goldberg RB, Holvey SM, Schneider J, the Glimepiride Study Group: A dose-response study of glimepiride in patients with NIDDM who have previously received sulfonylurea agents. *Diabetes Care* 19:849–856, 1996

Herrmann LS, Schersten B, Bitzen P-O, Kjellstrom T, Lindgarde F, Melander A: Therapeutic comparison of metformin and sulfonylurea, alone and in various combinations. *Diabetes Care* 20:1100–1109, 1997

Lebovitz HE: Alpha-glucosidase inhibitors. *Endocrinol Metab Clin North Am* 26:539–551, 1997

Meriden T: Progress with thiazolidinediones in the management of type 2 diabetes mellitus. *Clin Ther* 26:177–190, 2004

Misbin RI, Green L, Stadel BU, Gweriguian JL, Gubbi A, Flemming GA: Lactic acidosis in patients with diabetes treated with metformin. *N Engl J Med* 338:265–266, 1998

Raptis SA, Dimitriadis GD: Oral hypoglycemic agents: insulin secretagogues, alpha-glucosidase inhibitors and insulin sensitizers. *Exp Clin Endocrinol Diabetes* 109 (Suppl. 2):S265–S287, 2001

Riddle MC, Rosenstock J, Gerich J, Insulin Glargine 4002 Study Investigators: The Treat-to-Target Trial: randomized addition of glargine or human NPH insulin to oral therapy of type 2 diabetic patients. *Diabetes Care* 26:3080–3086, 2003

Schwartz S, Raskin P, Fonseca U, Graveline JF: Effect of troglitazone in insulin-treated patients with type 2 diabetes. *N Engl J Med* 338:861–866, 1998

Setter SM, Iltz JL, Thams J, Campbell RK: Metformin hydrochloride in the treatment of type 2 diabetes mellitus: a clinical review with a focus on dual therapy. *Clin Ther* 25:2991–3026, 2003

Shank ML, DelPrato S, DeFronzo RA: Bedtime insulin/daytime glipizide: effective therapy for sulfonylurea failures in NIDDM. *Diabetes* 44:165–172, 1995

Simonsen DC, Kourides IA, Feinglos M, Shamoon H, Fischette CT, Glipizide Gastrointestinal System Study Group: Efficacy, safety, and dose-response characteristics of glipizide gastrointestinal therapeutic system on glycemic control and insulin secretion in NIDDM. *Diabetes Care* 20:597–606, 1997

United Kingdom Prospective Diabetes Study (UKPDS) Group: Intensive blood-glucose control with sulphonylureas or insulin compared with conventional treatment and risk of complications in patients with type 2 diabetes (UKPDS 33). *Lancet* 352:837–853, 1998

United Kingdom Prospective Diabetes Study 16: Overview of 6 years' therapy of type II diabetes: a progressive disease. *Diabetes* 44:1249–1258, 1995

Zimmerman BR: Sulfonylureas. *Endocrinol Metab Clin North Am* 26:511–522, 1997

ASSESSMENT OF TREATMENT EFFICACY

In clinical practice, response to the treatment of type 2 diabetes mellitus should be monitored through a schedule of patient interviews and examinations with a comprehensive assessment of

- continued patient acceptance of the treatment plan and goals
- symptoms
- weight
- blood pressure
- smoking
- screening evaluations for complications, including
  - lipid levels
  - urine microalbumin-to-creatinine ratio
  - dilated eye exams
  - comprehensive foot exams
- various parameters of glycemic control

Among these parameters, glycemic control is unique in that techniques have been developed to allow both the patient and the health care team to independently and synergistically assess the response of glucose metabolism to therapy. This section will focus on assessment of treatment efficacy as reflected in glycemic targets (Table 3.13). In general, providers assess blood glucose control with assays for A1C. Intermittent measurements of fasting, preprandial, and postprandial plasma glucose levels in the office may be useful.

For most patients, SMBG is critical in that it creates a situation in which the patients can be in control of their own therapy. If patients are aware of the

---

Table 3.13 Glycemic Control for People with Diabetes

A1C	<7.0%*
Preprandial plasma glucose	90–130 mg/dl (5.0–7.2 mmol/l)
Postprandial plasma glucose†	<180 mg/dl (<10.0 mmol/l)

Key concepts in setting glycemic goals:
- Goals should be individualized.
- Certain populations (children, pregnant women, and elderly) require special considerations.
- Less intensive glycemic goals may be indicated in patients with severe or frequent hypoglycemia.
- More stringent glycemic goals (i.e., a normal A1C, <6%) may further reduce complications at the cost of increased risk of hypoglycemia (particularly in those with type 1 diabetes).
- Postprandial glucose may be targeted if A1C goals are not met despite reaching preprandial glucose goals.

*Referenced to a nondiabetic range of 4.0–6.0% using a DCCT-based assay.
†Postprandial glucose measurements should be made 1–2 h after the beginning of the meal, when levels generally peak in people with diabetes.

glycemic targets associated with the outcomes they seek to achieve, SMBG provides a way for them to critically evaluate their response to therapy and to assure themselves that they are reaching their goals. In this process, it is essential that patients and practitioners agree on mutually acceptable glycemic targets, the frequency and pattern of SMBG, and a plan for interpreting and acting on the results obtained.

To this end, it is generally useful for patients to keep a daily diary of their SMBG results, not only so that they can periodically assess their results, but also so they can share them with the health care team. Sometimes recording food intake, activity, symptoms, and doses of diabetes medications simultaneously provides the patient and health care team with a better understanding of the factors that influence the level of glycemic control.

The frequency and type of monitoring of diabetes therapy should be determined in consultation with patients, taking into account the nature of their diabetes, their overall treatment plans and goals, and their abilities. The practitioner should also be aware of the financial burden of SMBG supplies, which can be the limiting factor for compliance with recommended blood glucose monitoring, although meters and tests strips are a covered benefit for most insured patients. A comprehensive list of products available for diabetes care, including SMBG, can be found in the American Diabetes Association's *Buyer's Guide to Diabetes Products*, an annual supplement to *Diabetes Forecast*. Although SMBG requires a modicum of manual dexterity, cooperation, and intelligence, with currently available equipment and patient education, almost everyone can successfully monitor their blood glucose.

Each of the assessment methods described below has advantages and disadvantages. Most often, a combination of methods is used to determine the degree of metabolic control.

OFFICE METHODS

At office visits, clinicians can assess the degree of blood glucose control with a laboratory venous plasma glucose determination, capillary plasma glucose determination, and/or an assay for A1C. These measurements are of value in different ways. The venous glucose or capillary glucose is an index of moment-to-moment control and can also be used to compare with simultaneously obtained patient SMBG results to check the patient's technique as well as the meter's accuracy. A1C concentration reflects the level of glucose control for the preceding 2–3 months and has been well established through the DCCT, the UKPDS, and other prospective studies to predict the risk of developing complications. Other glycated serum proteins can be measured in the laboratory but are not as well validated to reflect risk of complications. Each reflects the level of glycemic control over shorter periods of time proportional to their circulating half-life.

Office Glucose Determinations

Fasting as well as 1- to 2-h postprandial glucose levels are easily measured and useful parameters for determining metabolic control. The major drawback to random plasma glucose determinations, particularly in a patient with moderate to severe disease, is that it is difficult to know what a single blood glucose determination reflects other than the level of glucose at that moment. Blood glucose levels can range widely during the day, so random determinations may represent peak values, trough values, or values in between. Furthermore, if the patient is visiting the office because of intercurrent illness, blood glucose levels will be of little value in determining overall glycemic control because illness generally alters glucose tolerance. Also, some patients become more conscientious about following prescribed therapy just before office visits, in which case the random plasma glucose level may be misleadingly low. For these reasons, plasma or capillary blood glucose levels should be supplemented at regular intervals with an A1C assay.

A1C

Glycated hemoglobin is expressed as a percentage of total hemoglobin, i.e., the fraction of total hemoglobin that has glucose attached. Depending on the assay method and laboratory used, the test may be called glycohemoglobin, glycated hemoglobin, glycosylated hemoglobin, hemoglobin A_1, or hemoglobin A_{1c}. Although the different measurements all have different normal ranges, the results of all assay methods, when properly performed, correlate closely with each other. Efforts are underway to standardize these methods worldwide. Clinicians should become familiar with the assay used in their clinical laboratory, the factors that can interfere with it, and the normal range and should be vigilant for changes in the assay methodology used by the laboratories that they employ. These tests are generally referred to as A1C with a normal range of 4–6%.

An A1C may be used to assess the effects of changes in therapy made 4–12 weeks earlier. It should not be used to determine the need for short-term changes in treatment. Blood glucose levels, generally from SMBG, are still the best means by which hour-to-hour and day-to-day changes in insulin management can be determined. However, health care providers have learned not to rely solely on SMBG results because the measurements are subject to errors in technique and the records are subject to errors of omission and commission.

Certain conditions and interfering substances affect A1C results, depending on the assay method used. Any condition that increases erythrocyte turnover, e.g., bleeding, pregnancy, or hemolysis, will spuriously lower A1C concentration in all assays. In addition, hemoglobinopathies, e.g., sickle cell trait or disease or hemoglobin C or D, will falsely lower results when hemoglobins are separated by nonspecific methods based on charge, solubility, and size. Other conditions, e.g., uremia, high concentrations of fetal hemoglobin (HbF), high aspirin doses (usually >10 g/day), or high concentrations of ethanol, may falsely increase A1C levels. These artifacts do not occur in all methods, and specific reference to the manufacturer's package insert for the test assay used is the best guide to a particular assay's performance in various clinical situations.

However, although the assay reflects glycemic control over the preceding 2–3 months, the result is time-weighted in that the level of glycemic control over the past month is a much greater determinant of the result than the previous months. Therefore, the A1C test is fairly useful in assessing trends in response to therapy over a period as short as a month.

In general, well-controlled patients with type 2 diabetes and stable courses of treatment who perform SMBG should have their A1C determined at least twice a year. More frequent monitoring of A1C can be useful in assessing the response to therapy in patients with unstable courses of treatment or changes in therapy, in patients on insulin therapy, and in those not achieving glycemic control goals.

PATIENT MONITORING

Between office visits, patients can determine their degree of metabolic control by performing SMBG, and other tests as needed, and keeping records of results.

Blood Glucose Checks

With the advent of SMBG and the availability of multiple pharmaceutical classes of drugs that attack the pathophysiology of diabetes in different areas, near-normal glucose levels have become a realistic goal for many individuals with diabetes. Although in clinical trials SMBG has not been demonstrated to change outcomes in type 2 diabetes management when evaluated in isolation, many diabetes self-management training programs have been shown to help reduce complications (e.g., DIGAMI and Kumamoto studies). In all of these, SMBG was an integral part of the process, suggesting that SMBG is at least a component of effective therapy. Blood glucose monitoring is considerably more sensitive than urine glucose tests for the detection of hyperglycemia and provides the ability to detect hypoglycemia before it becomes symptomatic. SMBG, when combined with robust patient education, actively involves patients in the treatment process by allowing the patient to make adjustments in diet, exercise, and medication to achieve mutually agreed-upon targets. In the absence of periodic SMBG, it is almost impossible for patients to assess their response to the many activities that the health care team asks them to perform (e.g., nutritional changes, increased physical activity, taking medications as prescribed). SMBG is an extraordinarily valuable tool in the education process to help ensure patient commitment to the therapeutic plan.

It is critical that patients learn what to do with their SMBG results and have a well-established, concrete plan for action based on out-of-target results. Unfortunately, many patients faithfully perform frequent SMBG, record the results as instructed, and hand over results at semi-annual visits, not having been taught to look for trends in their numbers or use their results to assess the impact of their daily choices on glycemic control. Patients who understand the relationship between medications, food, and activity and their glucose levels and who learn to spot trends are better able to meet glucose targets or ask for assistance between visits.

SMBG is recommended for all patients on insulin or insulin secretagogues and sulfonylureas, because it allows for the identification of minimal and/or asymptomatic episodes of hypoglycemia. Recurrent mild or asymptomatic hypoglycemia is a very strong risk factor for severe hypoglycemia. Although severe hypoglycemia is relatively rare in type 2 diabetes, it can have devastating consequences, such as trauma as a result of confusion or loss of consciousness. It is also commonly accepted that mild or unrecognized hypoglycemia is part of the reason why patients treated with insulin or a sulfonylurea have a proclivity for weight gain. Therefore, it is essential to have patients critically assess the nature of any "hypoglycemic" symptoms that occur during the day. Many patients are fearful or overconcerned about hypoglycemia and routinely consume extra calories when they are hungry, sweaty, nervous, or upset because they believe that they are hypoglycemic. Monitoring generally documents that most symptoms in patients with type 2 diabetes are not related to hypoglycemia and should not be treated with food.

SMBG is also useful for patients at the early stages of type 2 diabetes treated with nutrition and physical activity, because it allows for day-to-day determination of the adequacy of their efforts. Furthermore, it gives patients the opportunity to assess glycemic excursions and contact the health care team early, if necessary, with deteriorations in glycemic control during periods of stress, such as those caused by infection or trauma.

Timing of SMBG will vary depending on the diabetes therapy. Useful times to monitor include fasting (in the morning before breakfast to assess basal glycemia), before meals and at bedtime (to assess the risk of hypoglycemia), 1–2 h after meals (to assess the maximal excursion in glucose during the day), in the middle of the sleep cycle (to assess whether there is any nocturnal hypoglycemia, which can be asymptomatic), and when experiencing symptoms (such as "hypoglycemic spells" or illness). It is important not to allow patients to get into the rut of only checking at one particular time of day. There are rare individuals in whom only a certain time of day is associated with abnormal results, and in those, more focused monitoring at that time of day may be appropriate. For some patients, their highest blood glucose of the day will be the fasting glucose or 1–2 h after breakfast. For others, their highest levels will be at another time of day depending on eating habits and activity.

Likewise, there are significant numbers of patients who have near-normal levels of premeal glucose who have substantial hyperglycemic responses to meals, particularly in the context of low-fat meal plans. Both in the setting of gestational diabetes and in well-controlled type 2 diabetes, 1-h postprandial capillary blood glucose levels have correlated more strongly with A1C than fasting or premeal glucose levels. Patients with near-normal 1-h postprandial glucose levels clearly have excellent overall glucose control.

Some clinicians have patients concentrate on premeal glucose levels if the results are generally in the high 100s or higher. Once the premeal glucose levels reach the middle to low 100s, the patients switch to targeting 1- to 2-h postprandial glucose levels, because that amplifies the effects of lifestyle issues on glycemia and allows patients to identify how moderate changes in meal plan, activity, and medications have a significant impact on glycemic control. Even after substantial inappropriate changes in food intake, activity, or timing or dose of medication, blood glucose values often return to near-normal levels overnight or by the time of the next meal. Targeting therapy to SMBG results at just one time of day could leave the patient with a less than ideal overall response to therapy.

The frequency of SMBG should be matched to individual patient needs and treatment. Most clinicians ask patients who take hypoglycemic agents to monitor at least once a day, varying before meals and bedtime and at mid-sleep, as well as when they have hypoglycemic symptoms. Some ask insulin-treated patients to monitor much more frequently (≥4 times/day). In the subset of patients who achieve stable blood glucose levels, it is generally appropriate to decrease the frequency of SMBG to a few times a week, again concentrating on postprandial glucose levels. It is critical that SMBG be frequent enough that the patient and provider have a good understanding of both the adequacy of the treatment regimen and the stability of glycemic control.

There is a wide assortment of meters available with many different features that may be very important to individual patients. The meters come in various shapes and sizes, from the size of a pen to a card to a small box. Most have some memory for previous results, and some have sophisticated features that allow the user to record medication doses and symptoms. Use of meters that still require the strip to be wiped or blotted is not recommended, as that provides an extra step in which poor technique can affect results.

Some use significantly smaller sample volumes than others, which may be an advantage for patients who have difficulty obtaining an adequate drop. Newer meters allow sampling from sites, such as the forearm. This can be very helpful to patients who have in the past used fingertips exclusively for monitoring and have scarring and pain with fingertip sampling. Some devices allow the user to wipe on blood and/or redose the strip if an inadequate volume of blood is applied to the strip initially. As a result, some meters are clearly much easier to use than others, especially for patients with physical or cognitive impairments. Several can be adapted to voice synthesizers that provide audio output of results. The use of an automated lancing device for fingersticks is recommended. Several models are available: some more suited to children, those who frequently monitor, or the squeamish.

The bulk of the expense of SMBG is in the strips. It is generally possible for most patients to get a meter heavily discounted or for free. The role of the diabetes educator in helping patients determine which meter meets their needs and the role of vendors in minimizing the financial repercussions of SMBG are critical in making this technique as widely and appropriately applied as possible.

Urine Glucose Determinations

The determination of urine glucose has, for the most part, been superseded by SMBG. Urine glucose measurements are indirect and imprecise, and they should be reserved for patients who cannot or will not check blood glucose levels. The average renal threshold for glucose is ~180 mg/dl (~10 mmol/l), but it can vary widely between patients and even in the same patient over time. A normal urine glucose cannot distinguish between hypoglycemia, euglycemia, or moderate hyperglycemia.

Urine Ketone Determinations

Patients with type 2 diabetes rarely have ketosis. However, some experts recommend home ketone testing in the presence of serious illness. Positive nonfasting urine ketones in a patient with type 2 diabetes is a worrisome finding that requires further evaluation.

Patient Records

The patient should be encouraged to record SMBG determinations in tabular form, so that glycemic levels at various times of the day can be scanned visually with ease. Some meters contain memories that can be downloaded into a computer to produce such glucose logs. Generally, writing down glucose levels is still preferable because it allows patients to more frequently critically assess the pattern of glucose levels over time. On a long-term basis, the burden of keeping detailed logs of glucose monitoring, food intake, doses of diabetes medications, activity, symptoms (physical as well as emotional, including their circumstance and treatment), and the relative timing of all these parameters is generally more than most patients are willing to accept. Used intermittently, these kinds of records are invaluable in assessing how various lifestyle issues and therapeutic efforts interact in determining hour-to-hour and day-to-day changes in glycemic control. They are critical in developing lifestyle plans (diet and exercise) with patients and can serve to reinforce positive behaviors and to demonstrate their beneficial outcomes.

Patient records are also helpful to the health care team because they indicate the patient's degree of interest in control and provide information necessary for development of effective therapeutic plans. Almost all patients willing to keep records should be able to achieve excellent glycemic control, as they are clearly both willing and able to make substantial efforts in their self-care behavior. Furthermore, the records are usually invaluable in providing guidance about where to concentrate efforts in trying to improve glycemic control.

BIBLIOGRAPHY

American Diabetes Association: Standards of medical care in diabetes (Position Statement). *Diabetes Care* 27 (Suppl. 1):S15–S35, 2004

Dagogo JS, Santiago JV: Pathophysiology of type 2 diabetes and modes of action of therapeutic interventions. *Arch Intern Med* 157:1802–1817, 1997

deVeciana M, Major CA, Morgan MA, Asrat T, Toohey JS, Lien JM, Evans AT: Postprandial versus preprandial blood glucose monitoring in women with gestational diabetes mellitus requiring insulin therapy. *N Engl J Med* 333:1237–1241, 1995

Faas A, Schellevis FG, van Eijk JTM: The efficacy of self-monitoring of blood glucose in NIDDM subjects: a criteria-based review of the literature. *Diabetes Care* 20:1482–1486, 1997

Franz MJ: Lifestyle modifications for diabetes management. *Endocrinol Metab Clin North Am* 26:499–510, 1997

Goldstein DE, Little RR: Monitoring glycemia in diabetes: short-term assessment. *Endocrinol Metab Clin North Am* 26:475–486, 1997

Malmberg K, Ryden L, Efendic S, Herlitz J, Nicol P, Waldenstrom A, Wedel H, Welin L, on Behalf of the DIGAMI Study Group: Randomized trial of insulin-glucose infusion followed by subcutaneous insulin treatment in diabetic patients with acute myocardial infarction (DIGAMI study): effects on mortality at 1 year. *J Am Coll Cardiol* 26:57–65, 1995

Ohkubo Y, Kishikawa H, Araki E, Isami S, Motoyoshi S, Kojima Y, Furuyoshi N, Shichiri M: Intensive insulin therapy prevents the progression of diabetic microvascular complications in Japanese patients with non-insulin-dependent diabetes mellitus: a randomized prospective 6-year study. *Diabetes Res Clin Pract* 28:103–117, 1995

Special Therapeutic Situations

Highlights

Pregnancy

Diabetes in Youth
Differentiating Type 1 and Type 2 Diabetes in Youth
Screening for Type 2 Diabetes in Youth
Treating Type 2 Diabetes in Youth

Hospitalized, Surgical, and Critically Ill Patients

Hyperosmolar Hyperglycemic State
Pathophysiology
Therapy
Identification and Treatment of Precipitating Causes
Risks of Aggressive Treatment

Highlights
Special Therapeutic Situations

PREGNANCY

■ Glycemic control immediately before conception and during pregnancy is critical. Narrower glycemic targets help assure the health of both mother and developing child. Plasma glucose targets are 60–90 mg/dl (3.5–5.0 mmol/l) fasting and <120 mg/dl (<6.7 mmol/l) postprandial.

■ Insulin should be used during pregnancy when dietary management fails to keep blood glucose levels within target ranges.

■ A team with experience in the care of this high-risk group should care for the pregnant woman with diabetes.

DIABETES IN YOUTH

■ Young people with new-onset type 2 diabetes are often obese, inactive, and have a strong family history of type 2 diabetes.

■ The presence of ketoacidosis does not rule out the presence of type 2 diabetes in children.

■ Metformin is the only approved oral medication for type 2 diabetes in children.

■ Insulin should be used in children who have metabolic decompensation or who do not achieve adequate control with diet, exercise, or metformin therapy.

■ Young people with type 2 diabetes have a high risk for cardiovascular disease and should be treated aggressively for hypertension, dyslipidemia, and nephropathy.

HOSPITALIZED, SURGICAL, AND CRITICALLY ILL PATIENTS

■ Intravenous insulin decreases mortality in individuals with diabetes in the intensive care unit and in those who have suffered a myocardial infarction.

■ Care of the critically ill individual with type 2 diabetes should be via a collaboration of nursing, nutrition, and pharmacy units as well as the medical staff and patient. Institutional protocols should be developed and staff trained to allow strict glycemic control.

- Goals of therapy are <110 mg/dl (<6.1 mmol/l) preprandial and <180 mg/dl (<10.0 mmol/l) postprandial in hospitalized patients and 80–110 mg/dl (4.4–6.1 mmol/l) in critically ill surgical patients.

HYPEROSMOLAR HYPERGLYCEMIC STATE

- Hyperosmolar hyperglycemic state (HHS) is characterized by markedly elevated plasma glycose levels, dehydration, and hyperosmolality usually with an absence of significant ketoacidosis. Ketonuria can be detected in a portion of individuals.

- HHS usually develops slowly in elderly or incapacitated individuals and presents with significant dehydration, oliguria, hypotension, and altered mental status.

- Therapy is directed toward replacement of lost fluids and electrolytes and administration of insulin.

Special Therapeutic Situations

PREGNANCY

Pregnancy presents a challenge, with potential clinical difficulties, for both the woman with preexisting diabetes and her unborn baby. The fetus/newborn of a mother with diabetes has an increased risk of death, prematurity, and morbidity, e.g., congenital defects, macrosomia, hypoglycemia, hypocalcemia, hyperbilirubinemia, respiratory distress syndrome. The mother with diabetes faces an increased risk of acceleration of microvascular complications involving the kidneys and eyes, particularly if hypertension is present.

Diabetic pregnancy should be planned so that conception occurs when the patient has near-normal plasma glucose levels and glycated hemoglobin A_{1c} (A1C) values within the normal range for pregnancy. After conception, treatment should not only continue to achieve glycemic goals, but also meet the nutritional requirements of the fetus. Although several recent studies have suggested that both sulfonylureas and metformin are relatively safe and effective in treating gestational diabetes, it is recommended that oral diabetes medications be discontinued and the patient switched to insulin therapy before conception. A patient being treated with oral agents who becomes pregnant should begin insulin therapy.

The physician should inform the patient of the risks to her health and that of the baby. Because the risks of pregnancy complicated by diabetes are great and involve both mother and fetus/newborn and the treatment program is complex, based on multiple injections of insulin or use of the insulin pump with the goal of euglycemic regulation, care should involve appropriate specialists. Consultation with a physician skilled in the care of pregnant women with diabetes should be sought before conception or as soon as pregnancy is diagnosed to achieve normalization of blood glucose levels. Plasma glucose goals for women with diabetes during pregnancy are

- fasting 60–90 mg/dl (3.5–5.0 mmol/l)
- postprandial <120 mg/dl (<6.7 mmol/l)

The care of a pregnant woman with diabetes is best accomplished by an experienced health care team. The physician who assumes responsibility for such a patient must be completely familiar with proper management of the patient and her fetus/newborn during pregnancy, peripartum, and postpartum. The same vigorous attention to glycemic regulation and proper management of the patient and her fetus/newborn must be given to the individual who develops gestational diabetes during the second or third trimester.

BIBLIOGRAPHY

American Diabetes Association: *Medical Management of Pregnancy Complicated by Diabetes.* Jovanovic L, Ed. Alexandria, VA, American Diabetes Association, 2000

Kitzmiller JL, Buchanan TA, Kjos S, Combs CA, Ratner RE: Preconception care of diabetes, congenital malformations, and spontaneous abortions. *Diabetes Care* 19:514–541, 1996

DIABETES IN YOUTH

The pathophysiology of type 2 diabetes in young individuals is likely very similar to that seen in adults, with obesity and physical inactivity the primary inciting factors. Given the direct relationship between weight gain and the risk for diabetes, it is not surprising that the recent rise in obesity in young people is paralleled by an increase in the number of cases of type 2 diabetes. At least 15% of adolescents are defined as overweight and the incidence is rising, especially among minority children. In some communities, obesity rates are 33–50% and the incidence of type 2 diabetes is surpassing type 1 diabetes as the primary cause of diabetes in children. The increase in obesity in youth is related to both decreases in physical activity and consumption of food of high caloric density. In the U.S. 27% of high school boys and 43% of high school girls are estimated to undergo an insufficient amount of physical activity. Leisure-time physical activity decreases with age and is directly related to time spend viewing television. Studies have also demonstrated a correlation between television viewing and consumption of high-energy foods, further contributing to obesity.

DIFFERENTIATING TYPE 1 AND TYPE 2 DIABETES IN YOUTH

In the adolescent, type 2 diabetes can be differentiated from type 1 diabetes by the presence of significant obesity, the absence of islet cell antibodies, and normal or elevated fasting C-peptide levels. In many instances, there will be acanthosis nigricans and there is usually a significant family history of type 2 diabetes. The young person with type 2 diabetes typically does not present with significant weight loss but commonly has ketonuria, or even ketoacidosis. It has been suggested that the onset of puberty in obese children may be an inciting event for the development of diabetes in this susceptible population.

SCREENING FOR TYPE 2 DIABETES IN YOUTH

The American Diabetes Association and the American Academy of Pediatrics recommend screening at age >10 years or at onset of puberty, if earlier, for children who have body mass index (BMI) >85th percentile and any of the following risk factors:

- a first- or second-degree relative who has diabetes
- at-risk race/ethnic group
- signs of insulin resistance, such as acanthosis nigricans, hypertension, polycystic ovary syndrome, or dyslipidemia

Screening can be via measurement of fasting plasma glucose or by performing a 2-h oral glucose tolerance test. Follow-up testing should be performed every 2 years in at-risk patients.

TREATING TYPE 2 DIABETES IN YOUTH

The approach to treatment of pediatric type 2 diabetes is complicated by the fact that there are few data comparing the relative efficacies of diet, exercise, insulin, and other drug therapies in this population. However, given the early onset of type 2 diabetes, aggressive therapies are required given the longer diabetes duration and subsequent risk for macrovascular and microvascular complications. An aggressive intervention directed toward weight loss, including dietary restriction and exercise, along with an educational plan that includes the primary caregivers, is an essential part of the therapeutic plan.

Goals of treatment in this population include the achievement of near-normal glycemic control (A1C <7%) to eliminate symptoms of hyperglycemia and stem development of microvascular and macrovascular complications. Exogenous insulin has traditionally been used to treat childhood diabetes, and this should be instituted in individuals with significantly elevated glucose levels and in anyone demonstrating ketosis. Early administration of insulin may increase compliance, perhaps by conveying a message about the significance of the disease.

Although many oral agents are available to treat type 2 diabetes in adults and all have been used in children, metformin is the only oral drug approved by the U.S. Food and Drug Administration to treat type 2 diabetes in children. Metformin can decrease A1C by ~1% in this population. Sulfonylureas are effective in adults but are associated with hypoglycemia and weight gain and therefore should not be used as first-line agents. Although theoretically attractive because of their insulin-sensitizing effect, the thiazolidinedione class of medications has not been extensively studied in the pediatric population; ongoing studies will clarify their use.

As in adults, dyslipidemia and hypertension should be treated aggressively, and cessation of smoking is a critical component of care. Screening and treatment with angiotensin-converting enzyme inhibitors for microalbuminuria should be part of the treatment plan. Hypertension treatment should be individualized based on age, height, and sex of the patient. The National Cholesterol Education Program lipid guidelines for children regard the following levels as desirable: LDL cholesterol <110 mg/dl, HDL cholesterol >45 mg/dl, and triglyceride <125 mg/dl. The American Diabetes Association has recently proposed that children with diabetes have a target LDL cholesterol level <100 mg/dl. Dietary lipid management along with niacin and cholestyramine treatment are the initial therapy options. Recent studies with statins suggest that they are safe and effective in children.

BIBLIOGRAPHY

American Diabetes Association: Management of dyslipidemia in children and adolescents with diabetes. *Diabetes Care* 26:2194–2197, 2003

American Diabetes Association: Screening for type 2 diabetes (Position Statement). *Diabetes Care* 27 (Suppl. 1):S11–S14, 2004

Aye T, Levitsky LL: Type 2 diabetes: an epidemic disease in childhood. *Curr Opin Pediatr* 15:411–415, 2003

Bloomgarden ZT: Type 2 diabetes in the young: the evolving epidemic. *Diabetes Care* 27:998–1010, 2004

Kaufman FR: Type 2 diabetes mellitus in children and youth: a new epidemic. *J Pediatr Endocrinol Metab* 15 (Suppl. 2):737–744, 2002

Ogden CL, Carroll MD, Flegal KM: Epidemiologic trends in overweight and obesity. *Endocrinol Metab Clin North Am* 32:741–760, 2003

Rosenbloom AL, Silverstein JH: *Type 2 Diabetes in Children & Adolescents.* Alexandria, VA, American Diabetes Association, 2003

HOSPITALIZED, SURGICAL, AND CRITICALLY ILL PATIENTS

Numerous observational studies as well as two randomized, prospective trials that used intravenous insulin therapy have revolutionized thinking about postoperative and inpatient care of diabetes and hyperglycemia. They found that intensive insulin treatment of critically ill hospitalized patients reduces mortality without increasing morbidity due to hypoglycemia. In the first study, patients presenting with acute myocardial infarction were randomized to intravenous infusion of insulin (containing potassium chloride), which was titrated to achieve glucose levels of 126–180 mg/dl (7.0–10.0 mmol/l). After discharge from the intensive care unit (ICU), patients randomized to insulin infusion were treated with multiple daily injections of insulin. The second trial demonstrated that intravenous insulin infusion in the surgical ICU to achieve a target glucose 80–110 mg/dl (4.4–6.1 mmol/l) reduced the risk of in-hospital mortality in general, with a specific benefit of reducing the risk associated with infectious complications of prolonged ICU treatment.

Health care organizations, including the American Diabetes Association, now suggest that the treatment of diabetes and hyperglycemia in the hospital should target plasma glucose levels approaching normoglycemia:

- preprandial: <110 mg/dl (<6.1 mmol/l)
- peak postprandial: <180 mg/dl (<10.0 mmol/l)
- critically ill surgical patients: 80–110 mg/dl (4.4–6.1 mmol/l)

Achieving such levels of glycemic control in the hectic inpatient environment presents a challenge to patients, health care providers, and health care systems and requires the collaboration of the nursing, nutrition, and pharmacy units as well as medical staff and patients. Institutional protocols should be developed and staff trained to allow these levels of control to be achieved. Preprinted order sets facilitate adherence to protocols, and numerous examples are available in the literature.

Most authorities advocate intravenous infusion of insulin instead of subcutaneous administration in the operating room and the ICU. To the extent that intravenous administration can be used elsewhere in the health care system, this makes it possible to carefully control the insulin delivery appropriately based on frequent measurement of blood glucose and changes in diet, other medications, and physical activity.

Unless the surgical condition is an emergency, the patient should be allowed sufficient time to achieve acceptable control of hyperglycemia before surgery. If possible, the patient should have a complete evaluation of metabolic state and thorough assessment of diabetic complications, including renal and cardiovascular disease, before surgery.

It is now possible for a patient with diabetes mellitus to undergo surgical operations with little more than normal risk, unless the operation is done under emergency conditions that do not allow complete evaluation and preparation of the patient. The objectives of management before, during, and after surgery are to prevent hypoglycemia, which can lead to coma, and to prevent excessive hyperglycemia and ketoacidosis, which can complicate postoperative care by increasing the risk of major infections, thrombosis, dehydration, excessive protein loss, and electrolyte imbalance. To accomplish these ends, the anesthetic technique (regional or general) and the anesthetic agent should disrupt metabolic control as little as possible. Special attention should be given to maintaining proper fluid and electrolyte balance and blood glucose levels. Patients with diabetes who have been treated with diet or oral agents may need insulin therapy for control of hyperglycemia during the acute stress period of a major surgical procedure.

To assume responsibility for the management of patients with type 2 diabetes during and after surgery, the clinician must learn specific techniques involved in preparing the patient for surgery and for managing the patient during and after the operation. The major principles governing the management of surgical candidates on the day of operation are presented in Table 4.1.

Table 4.1 Principles Governing Management of Patients with Diabetes During Hospitalization and Surgery

- Good metabolic control is associated with improved hospital outcomes. Target plasma glucose levels are <110 mg/dl (<6.1 mmol/l) preprandial and <180 mg/dl (<10.0 mmol/l) postprandial.
- Intensive insulin therapy with intravenous insulin, with the goal of maintaining blood glucose 80–110 mg/dl (4.4–6.1 mmol/l), reduces morbidity and mortality among critically ill patients in the surgical ICU.
- Intravenous insulin infusion is safe and effective for achieving metabolic control during major surgery, hemodynamic instability, and NPO status.
- Intravenous insulin infusion is safe and effective for patients who have poorly controlled diabetes and widely fluctuating blood glucose levels or who are insulin deficient or severely insulin resistant.
- Intravenous insulin infusion, followed by multidose subcutaneous insulin therapy, improves survival in patients with diabetes after myocardial infarction.
- For insulin-deficient patients, despite reductions or the absence of caloric intake, basal insulin must be provided to prevent diabetic ketoacidosis.
- Use of scheduled insulin improves blood glucose control compared with orders based on sliding-scale insulin coverage alone.
- For patients who are alert and demonstrate accurate insulin self-administration and glucose monitoring, insulin self-management should be allowed as an adjunct to standard nurse-delivered diabetes management.
- Patients with no prior history of diabetes who are found to have hyperglycemia (random blood glucose >125 mg/dl [>6.9 mmol/l]) during hospitalization should have follow-up testing for diabetes within 1 month of hospital discharge.
- Establishing a multidisciplinary team that sets and implements institutional guidelines, protocols, and standardized order sets for the hospital results in reduced hypoglycemic and hyperglycemic events.
- Diabetes education, medical nutrition therapy, and timely diabetes-specific discharge planning are essential components of hospital-based diabetes care.

From Clement et al.

BIBLIOGRAPHY

Alberti KGMM: Diabetes and surgery. In *Diabetes Mellitus: Theory and Practice.* 4th ed. Rifkin H, Porte D, Eds. New York, Elsevier, 1990, p. 626–633

Clement S, Braithwaite SS, Magee MF, Ahmann A, Smith EP, Schafer RG, Hirsch IB: Management of diabetes and hyperglycemia in hospitals. *Diabetes Care* 27:553–591, 2004

HYPEROSMOLAR HYPERGLYCEMIC STATE

PATHOPHYSIOLOGY

The hyperosmolar hyperglycemic state (HHS), also known as hyperglycemic hyperosmolar nonketotic coma (HHNC), is characterized by markedly elevated plasma glucose levels, dehydration, hyperosmolality, and, generally, absence of significant ketoacidosis. The presence of some ketonuria or mild ketonemia can be detected in a portion of the individuals. HHS occurs more frequently in the elderly and usually develops insidiously. It often presents with nervous system signs and symptoms from simple lethargy to coma and death. The depletion of fluids leads to hypotension and poor tissue perfusion, which can cause impairment of renal function, stroke, and other thromboembolic events.

The severe hyperglycemic state occurs due to a combination of inadequate control of glucose levels, defective concentrating ability of the kidney due to the presence of the glucose, and inability of the patient to respond to the hyperglycemic state by increasing fluid intake. Because elderly individuals have an intrinsic decline in renal function and may have an altered thirst center or other disabilities that prevent effective hydration, they are particularly vulnerable to the development of HHS.

Progressive elevation of the glucose levels often is triggered by infection or other stressors such as stroke or myocardial infarction. However, in many patients, there is no identifiable inciting event. The glucose remains largely in the extracellular space and shifts water osmotically from the intracellular compartment, which is then filtered through the kidney. This results in the development of glucosuric diuresis with loss of water and salt. The concentrating capacity of the kidney is disrupted due to the presence of glucose in the urine and can exacerbate fluid loss.

Normally, the rise in serum osmolality triggers fluid intake, which prevents significant rises in plasma glucose by maintaining renal blood flow and glucose excretion in the urine. However, the presence of renal disease and/or inadequate fluid intake as a result of impaired thirst, weakness, or incapacity results in exacerbation of the osmotic diuresis, further collapse of intravascular volume, further decline in renal perfusion, and a rapid rise in plasma glucose level, all resulting in HHS.

On presentation, the patient typically shows signs of significant dehydration, oligouria, hypotension, and altered mental status. The patient may be hypothermic. Blood glucose is elevated (typically >500 mg/dl [>28 mmol/l]), and serum osmolarity is increased. Serum osmolality can be calculated as

$$\text{osmolarity (mOsm/l)} = 2 \times [\text{sodium}]/18 + [\text{BUN}]/2.8 + [\text{ethanol}]/4.6$$

where the concentrations of glucose, BUN, and ethanol are in mg/dl, and the concentration of sodium is in mEq/l. Normal serum osmolarity is 290 ± 5 mOsm/l.

In HHS, the osmolarity is generally >350 mOsm/l and can exceed 400 mOsm/l. Serum sodium and potassium levels can be high, normal, or low and do not reflect total body levels, which are uniformly depleted. Significant ion gap acidosis is not normally found, but lactic acidosis can develop due to poor tissue perfusion, uremic acidosis due to renal insufficiency, or ketoacidosis due to impaired insulin secretion and exacerbated insulin resistance.

THERAPY

The pathophysiology of HHS is dehydration, lack of insulin, and electrolyte disturbances. Thus, initial therapy is directed at correcting these metabolic abnormalities. Uncontrolled diabetes can result in significant fluid losses (averaging 100–200 ml/kg). In patients with hyperosmolar hyperglycemia, the mean fluid loss at presentation is ~9 liters.

In most instances, intravenous (IV) fluids are administered rapidly to patients with HHS, generally as 1 liter normal saline solution over the first few minutes and 200–500 ml/h in subsequent hours as needed to correct hypotension. For individuals with a history of congestive heart failure, chronic or acute renal failure, severe hypotension, or significant pulmonary disease, invasive hemodynamic monitoring should be considered. Despite the excess of water losses over sodium, the measured sodium can be low because of osmotic effects of glucose. These osmotic effects can be corrected using the formula:

$$\text{corrected sodium concentration} = \text{measured [sodium]} + 0.016\,(\text{[glucose]} - 100)$$

where sodium is in mEq/l and glucose in mg/dl.

Severe hypertriglyceridemia, which is more often seen in diabetic ketoacidosis, can cause a false decrease in the serum sodium concentration by ~1.0 mEq/l at a serum lipid concentration of 460 mg/dl.

An estimate of the patient's water deficit can be calculated using the corrected sodium concentration:

$$\text{water deficit in liters} = 0.6\,(\text{body weight in kilograms}) \times (\text{corrected sodium concentration}/140)$$

Once the patient is normotensive, urinary losses should be replaced with one-half normal saline solution. One-half the calculated water deficit should be replaced as a 5% dextrose solution over the first 12–24 h and the remainder over the subsequent 24 h. Once the serum glucose level reaches 250 mg/dl, fluids should contain 5% dextrose, and therapy should be aimed at maintaining the serum glucose in the 150–250 mg/dl range for 24 h to allow slow equilibration of osmotically active substances across cell membranes.

The key to fluid management is vigilant monitoring and adjustment on a continuous basis. In many instances, this is best performed in an intensive care setting.

Insulin Replacement

The initial fluid resuscitation can have a significant impact on glucose levels via simple intravascular dilution and stimulation of a glucosuric diuresis. Failure of the plasma glucose level to decline by 75–100 mg/dl/h usually implies inadequate volume administration or impairment of renal function.

Patients with HHS have significant dehydration and poor skin perfusion; thus, IV insulin is significantly more effective than subcutaneous (SC) insulin. In cases where there is insufficient nursing monitoring or IV access to allow for safe IV administration, hourly intramuscular injections of regular insulin are an acceptable substitute. It is important that a needle of adequate length—at least 1.5 inches for adults—be used. An initial priming dose of 10 units IV insulin should be followed by a continuous infusion of 0.1 units/kg/h, with adjustments made on an hourly basis to bring the glucose level to ~250 mg/dl. At this point, 5% dextrose infusion should be starting while continuing IV insulin. Only after the patient is stabilized and eating can SC insulin can be initiated and the IV infusion of insulin be stopped. The glucose level should be checked in 2 h and at least every 4 h subsequently, until a relatively stable insulin regimen is determined. Early conversion to oral feeding and SC insulin therapy has been associated with shorter length of hospital stay. A proportion of patients with HHS do not require therapy for their diabetes after hospitalization, and most do not require insulin.

Electrolyte Replacement

In HHS, typical electrolyte deficits are as follows:

- sodium: 7–13 mEq/kg
- chloride: 3–7 mEq/kg
- potassium: 5–15 mEq/kg
- phosphate, as phosphorus: 70–140 mmol
- calcium: 50–100 mEq
- magnesium: 50–100 mEq

Sodium. Total body sodium is always decreased by osmotic diuresis due to glucosuria. Sodium losses are proportionally less than water losses and should be adequately replaced by the infusion of normal saline.

Potassium. Potassium losses during the development of HHS can be quite high (3–10 mEq/kg) but may be milder than that seen in DKA. The loss of potassium in HHS is secondary to osmotic diuresis, hyperaldosteronism (secondary hypotension), and the effect of protein catabolism. Serum potassium is usually normal or even high at presentation, but the initial therapy with fluids and insulin will cause the serum potassium level to fall. Potassium should be replaced in the first hours of treatment once urine output is adequate, the ECG shows no evidence of hyperkalemia, and the serum potassium level is <5 mEq/l. Replacement with potassium acetate, potassium phosphate, or a mixture of the two avoids administration of excess chloride.

In patients with renal insufficiency, early potassium replacement should still be indicated with frequent intense monitoring. Caution must be exercised in patients with diabetic nephropathy who may have renal tubular acidosis associated with hyperaldosteronism and hyporeninemia (and resultant hyperkalemia).

Other electrolytes. Hyperchloremia is common when chloride is given in equivalent amounts with sodium in the treatment of ketoacidosis. No specific therapy is advocated to correct chloride levels during the treatment of HHS. Phosphate is depleted in patients with HHS, but patients usually present with an elevated serum phosphate level that declines with therapy. No well-documented clinical benefit of phosphate administration has been demonstrated in the treatment of HHS, although most authorities recommend phosphate therapy, which can be administered as part of potassium replacement, with monitoring for its possible complications—hypocalcemia and hypomagnesemia.

Magnesium. As many as 40% of outpatients with diabetes and 90% of patients with uncontrolled diabetes after 12 h of therapy are hypomagnesemic. Manifestations of hypomagnesemia include ECG changes, arrhythmias, muscle weakness, convulsions, stupor, confusion, and agitation. Because it is predominantly intracellular, serum magnesium levels do not reflect total body stores. As with phosphate, no clinical trials have demonstrated a salutary effect of magnesium replacement in HHS. However, with symptoms consistent with low magnesium, the levels should be monitored and replaced to maintain magnesium levels in the normal range.

IDENTIFICATION AND TREATMENT OF PRECIPITATING CAUSES

Most of the mortality related to HHS is due to the underlying cause. At a minimum, all patients should be ruled out for myocardial infarction and carefully screened for infection by careful physical exam, chest X ray, and urinalysis, with consideration of empiric cultures and antibiotic therapy. In the obtunded patient and in those with altered mental status with localizing signs, an imaging procedure of the brain should be considered because of the prevalence of stroke and subdural hematoma in these patients. Intra-abdominal processes are often difficult to diagnose due to frequent increases in amylase or transaminases coupled with abdominal pain or abnormal abdominal exam. Note that these patients often exhibit a hypercoagulable state; pulmonary embolus should be considered, and at a minimum, prophylactic anticoagulant therapy should be administered to prevent deep venous thrombosis.

RISKS OF AGGRESSIVE TREATMENT

The potential for cerebral edema following rapid fluid administration and the rapid correction of plasma osmolarity should be a constant concern in individuals with significant increases in serum osmolarity. However, cerebral edema occurs almost exclusively in young patients who have nonhyperosmolar diabetes with diabetic ketoacidosis. This complication is exceedingly rare in adult patients with HHS. However, it is prudent to correct the hyperosmolar state over 24–48 h and to initially maintain glucose levels in the range of 200–250 mg/dl (11.1–13.9 mmol/l).

BIBLIOGRAPHY

Ennis ED, Stahl EJVB, Dreisberg RA: The hyperosmolar hyperglycemic syndrome. *Diabetes Rev* 2:115–126, 1994

Magee MF, Bhatt BA: Management of decompensated diabetes: diabetic ketoacidosis and hyperglycemic hyperosmolar syndrome. *Crit Care Clin* 17:75–106, 2001

Wachtel TJ, Silliman RA, Lamberton P: Predisposing factors for the diabetic hyperosmolar state. *Arch Intern Med* 147:499–512, 1987

Detection and Treatment
of Chronic Complications

Highlights

Rationale for Optimizing Glycemic Control
   in Type 2 Diabetes

Accelerated Macrovascular Disease
   Diabetes as a Cardiovascular Risk Factor
   Screening for Cardiovascular Disease
   Importance of Modifying Vascular Risk Factors
   Treatment of Cardiovascular Disease

Diabetic Retinopathy
   Stages of Diabetic Retinopathy
   Prevention of Retinopathy
   Treatment of Retinopathy

Diabetic Renal Disease
   Clinical Presentation of Nephropathy
   Conditions that Influence Renal Function
   Prevention and Treatment of Diabetic Renal Disease

Diabetic Foot Problems
   Causes of Diabetic Foot Problems
   Prevention of Foot Problems
   Treatment of Foot Problems

Neuropathic Conditions

Polyneuropathy
Autonomic Neuropathy
Other Varieties of Diabetic Neuropathy
Diagnosis and Treatment of Neuropathy

Highlights
Detection and Treatment
of Chronic Complications

■ Individuals with type 2 diabetes are highly susceptible to microvascular complications, including retinopathy, neuropathy, and nephropathy.

■ Individuals with type 2 diabetes are also susceptible to macrovascular complications, including cardiac disease and stroke. These complications are the primary cause of premature death in type 2 diabetes.

■ The high incidence of hypertension and dyslipidemia in patients with type 2 diabetes contributes to microvascular and macrovascular complications.

■ Aggressive control of glycemia and hypertension and smoking cessation reduce the risk of microvascular complications.

■ Aggressive control of glycemia, hypertension, and dyslipidemia and smoking cessation reduce the risk of macrovascular complications.

■ Continuous monitoring for development of and aggressive treatment of secondary complications can reduce the risk for blindness, renal failure, amputation, and cardiovascular disease.

Detection and Treatment of Chronic Complications

In the past, many clinicians considered type 2 diabetes a "mild" form of diabetes compared with type 1 diabetes because these patients tend to have less labile glucose profiles and can often be managed satisfactorily with nutrition and exercise therapy and oral agents, rather than with insulin. Consequently, "tight" glycemic control was not considered a necessary treatment goal. However, people with type 2 diabetes are afflicted with the same devastating litany of diabetes-specific long-term microvascular and neurologic complications as patients with type 1 diabetes (Table 5.1) and clearly have a significant increase in the risk of macrovascular complications. Several recent clinical trials have demonstrated that improved glycemic control in those with type 2 diabetes reduces their rate of microvascular diabetic complications and likely reduces the risk of macrovascular events as well.

The complications associated with diabetes—loss of vision, renal failure requiring dialysis or transplantation, amputations, heart attacks, strokes, and premature mortality—cause immense burden to patients and belie the notion that type 2 diabetes is mild. Because of the "silent" onset of type 2 diabetes in many, up to 50% of individuals already have complications at diagnosis. In addition, comorbid conditions such as hypertension and dyslipidemia markedly increase the risk of cardiovascular disease. Because type 2 diabetes accounts for >90% of diabetes in the United States, affecting >17 million people, treatment of the underlying disease and complications is a major burden to our health care system that will continue to grow as the population ages.

This section reviews the detection, prevention, and treatment of long-term diabetes microvascular (retinopathy, nephropathy, and neuropathy) and macrovascular (coronary, cerebrovascular, and peripheral) complications that accompany type 2 diabetes. Patient cases that illustrate proper diagnosis, prevention, and treatment of diabetic complications are presented.

Table 5.1 Chronic Complications Associated with Type 2 Diabetes Mellitus

Vascular Diseases

- Macrovascular
  - Accelerated coronary atherosclerosis
  - Accelerated cerebrovascular atherosclerosis
  - Accelerated peripheral vascular disease

- Microvascular
  - Retinopathy
  - Nephropathy

Neuropathy Syndromes and Outcomes

- Sensorimotor neuropathy
  - Symmetrical polyneuropathy, bilateral (lower > upper limbs)
    - Pain
    - Foot deformity
    - Ulceration
  - Mononeuropathy
  - Diabetic amyotrophy
  - Neuropathic cachexia

- Autonomic neuropathy
  - Gastroparesis
  - Diabetic diarrhea
  - Neurogenic bladder
  - Sexual dysfunction
  - Orthostatic hypotension

Mixed Vascular and Neuropathic Diseases

- Leg ulcers
- Foot ulcers

RATIONALE FOR OPTIMIZING GLYCEMIC CONTROL IN TYPE 2 DIABETES

A strong association between hyperglycemia and microvascular disease risk has emerged from intervention studies designed to assess whether improved glucose control delays the development and progression of retinopathy, nephropathy, and neuropathy in patients with either type 1 diabetes or type 2 diabetes. In type 2 diabetes, evidence supporting the role of hyperglycemia in the development of diabetic microvascular complications initially emerged in the Kumamoto study and was confirmed in the larger United Kingdom Prospective Diabetes Study (UKPDS). The UKPDS evaluated the effects of intensive blood glucose control with sulfonylurea, metformin, or insulin and less-intensive treatment with nutrition therapy, versus conventional treatment, on the risk of microvascular and macrovascular complications in patients newly diagnosed with type 2 diabetes. Over 10 years, glycated hemoglobin A_{1c} (A1C) averaged 7.0% in the intensive group compared with 7.9% in the conventionally treated group—an 11% reduction. There were no differences in A1C values among the patients randomized to either oral hypoglycemic agents or insulin therapy in the intensive treatment group. Compared to less-intensive therapy, intensive therapy reduced the risk by 12% for any diabetes-related end point. Most of this benefit was due to a 25% risk reduction in microvascular end points, including the need for retinal photocoagulation. These data strongly support the beneficial effects of effective antihyperglycemic therapy on the prevention of microvascular disease, regardless of the pathophysiology of the hyperglycemia.

Improved glycemic control also reduced the incidence of macrovascular complications in the UKPDS. There was a 16% risk reduction of myocardial infarction (MI) and sudden death, but diabetes-related mortality and all-cause mortality did not differ between the intensive and conventionally treated groups. A secondary randomization involved overweight patients with diabetes. In this substudy, patients treated with metformin, compared with the conventional group, had risk reductions of 32% for any diabetes-related end point, 42% for diabetes-related death, and 36% for all-cause mortality. There was an intermediate and statistically significant reduction when overweight patients were treated with insulin or sulfonylurea. Therefore, metformin therapy appears to decrease the risk of macrovascular disease in those with type 2 diabetes. Further studies are in progress to explore optimal treatment strategies for decreasing the excess cardiovascular disease risk in type 2 diabetes. Treatment should always be individualized, taking into consideration the patient's age and prognosis.

ACCELERATED MACROVASCULAR DISEASE

In the patient with diabetes, atherosclerosis involving the coronary, cerebrovascular, and peripheral vessels occurs at an earlier age and with greater frequency than it does in people without diabetes and is responsible for 80% of the mortality in adults with diabetes. Thus, the clinician should be alert for signs and symptoms of accelerated atherosclerosis among patients with diabetes.

Screening for coronary vessel disease should be considered in subjects with cardiac symptoms; an abnormal resting ECG; evidence of peripheral or carotid occlusive disease; a sedentary lifestyle; age >35 years and plans to begin an exercise program; and two or more cardiovascular risk factors, such as dyslipidemia, hypertension, smoking, family history of premature coronary artery disease (age <55 years in male and <65 years in female first-degree relatives), and micro- or macroalbuminuria.

Early detection of complications is crucial so that appropriate treatment can be introduced before major morbidity or mortality occurs. Although many patients with diabetes experience the same symptoms of coronary, cerebral, and peripheral vascular disease as patients without diabetes, clinicians should be aware that neuropathy and other factors may alter symptoms in the patient with diabetes. At least a third of patients with diabetes with coronary disease have no or atypical anginal symptoms, such as exertional dyspnea, rather than exertional chest pain. In addition, cerebral manifestations of hypoglycemia may mimic transient ischemic attacks, and symptoms of neuropathy may need to be distinguished from symptoms of intermittent claudication.

DIABETES AS A CARDIOVASCULAR RISK FACTOR

Studies have shown consistently that patients with diabetes mellitus have an excess of cardiovascular complications compared with patients without diabetes. In the United States, for example, those with diabetes are two- to fourfold as likely as those without diabetes to die from coronary artery disease, and the average annual incidence of cardiovascular sequelae is increased at least twofold in patients with diabetes. The risk of MI in subjects with diabetes is equivalent to a non-diabetic subject who has already suffered an MI. Most important, the relative risk for cardiovascular disease in women with type 2 diabetes is three to four times greater than for women without diabetes. In addition, women with diabetes complicated by coronary vessel disease appear to be particularly at risk, emphasizing the need for aggressive management in this population.

Type 2 diabetes is an independent risk factor for macrovascular disease. In addition, common coexistent conditions, including hypertension, dyslipidemia (decreased HDL cholesterol, increased triglyceride, and alterations in LDL cholesterol particle size and number), hyperlipidemia (increased LDL cholesterol), hypercoagulability, and obesity are also risk factors. The pattern of obesity is important, with central fat distribution (waist-to-hip ratio >0.9 in men and >0.75 in women or, alternatively, a waist ≥40 inches in men and ≥35 inches in women) associated with dyslipidemia, hypertension, and increased prevalence of cardiovascular disease, independent of obesity. Other risk factors demonstrated in people without diabetes, such as smoking and lack of exercise, apply as well to people with type 2 diabetes. Finally, renal failure, retinopathy, cardiac autonomic neuropathy, and microalbuminuria are additional markers of increased cardiovascular risk.

SCREENING FOR CARDIOVASCULAR DISEASE

Diagnostic testing for coronary artery disease should be considered in subjects with either typical or atypical cardiac symptoms or an abnormal resting ECG. In such patients, the pretest probability of an abnormal test is sufficiently high that a stress test with imaging procedure such as stress echocardiography or nuclear stress imaging or a cardiac catheterization is appropriate. Screening for coronary artery disease using a symptom-limited stress test is recommended for those

- with evidence of peripheral or carotid occlusive disease
- who are considering beginning a strenuous exercise program who lead a sedentary lifestyle and are over age 35 years
- with two or more cardiovascular risk factors, such as dyslipidemia, hypertension, smoking, family history of premature coronary artery disease, or albuminuria

Note that a substantial portion of patients will have abnormal results, but that it has never been demonstrated that asymptomatic patients with coronary artery disease benefit from intervention.

IMPORTANCE OF MODIFYING VASCULAR RISK FACTORS

Lifestyle measures, including weight reduction and exercise for overweight and obese patients with type 2 diabetes, may be the most cost-effective and safest modes of therapy and should be included in all treatment regimens. Successful weight reduction via a nutritious diet with proper portion sizes will improve atherogenic lipid profiles, glucose intolerance, hypertension, and, of course, obesity.

Although most studies demonstrating the efficacy of reducing cardiovascular risk factors, such as hypertension and dyslipidemia, in preventing or ameliorating cardiovascular disease have been performed in populations without diabetes, evidence from several studies suggests that such interventions will similarly benefit those with type 2 diabetes. The cardiovascular benefits for individuals with type 2 diabetes of lowering blood pressure and LDL cholesterol were documented in the UKPDS and in diabetic subgroups from several major clinical trials. More recently, the Heart Protection Study demonstrated that in people with diabetes age >40 years with total cholesterol >135 mg/dl, LDL reductions of ~30% with simvastatin were associated with an ~25% reduction in coronary events, independent of baseline LDL levels, prior vascular disease, or type 1 or type 2 diabetes.

Aspirin Therapy

Low-dose aspirin was demonstrated to be effective in reducing MIs in subjects without diabetes in the Physician's Health Study and in multiple other studies. A meta-analysis of 145 controlled trials of antiplatelet therapy showed that both men and women with diabetes had a significant reduction in vascular events. The Early Treatment Diabetic Retinopathy Study demonstrated the safety of aspirin therapy in people with diabetes and retinopathy and also found a reduction in MI risk. As a result of these findings, the American Diabetes Association recommends aspirin therapy for all people with diabetes who have evidence of macrovascular disease and consideration of aspirin therapy for those who are age >40 years and at high risk because of family history, smoking, hypertension, albuminuria, obesity, and/or dyslipidemia, unless there is a contraindication. Enteric-coated aspirin in doses of 75–162 mg daily is recommended. Adjunctive therapy with clopidogrel should be considered in high-risk subjects or aspirin-intolerant patients. Aspirin should not be used in those under age 21 years due to the increased risk of Reye's syndrome.

Management of Hypertension

There is incontrovertible evidence that hypertension complicating diabetes increases the risk of microvascular complications, cardiovascular events, and death. Epidemiologic analyses have demonstrated that blood pressure levels >115/75 mmHg are associated with increased cardiovascular events and mortality in diabetes. Control of hypertension in individuals with diabetes reduces the development and progression of coronary heart disease events, stroke, and nephropathy. Treatment of hypertension in those with diabetes should be vigorous.

The UKPDS explored the benefits of blood pressure lowering with captopril or atenolol on microvascular and macrovascular end points in subjects with type 2 diabetes and found that a 10/5 mmHg systolic/diastolic blood pressure reduction lowered the incidence of microvascular complications by 37%. Major cardiovascular events, including death, were reduced by 32%. In this study, the greatest benefits were observed in subjects achieving both glycemic *and* hypertension control. These results have been duplicated in more than a half-dozen studies using thiazide diuretics, angiotensin-converting enzyme (ACE) inhibitors, angiotensin-receptor blockers (ARBs), β-blockers, and calcium-channel blockers. No consistent differences in outcomes emerged between the different therapeutic agents listed.

Current recommendations are outlined in Table 5.2. Before initiating therapy, hypertension should be confirmed by repeat measurements. Automated ambulatory blood pressure monitoring may be especially helpful in people with diabetes, who often experience nocturnal blood pressure reduction. Autonomic dysfunction and orthostatic hypotension in individuals with long-standing diabetes or with symptoms should be excluded by measuring supine, sitting, and standing blood pressure. In individuals with mild hypertension (130–139/80–89 mmHg), a short trial of lifestyle modification may be tried, including weight reduction, increased exercise, smoking cessation, and reduced alcohol and sodium intake. Institute pharmacological therapy if these interventions fail.

Pharmacotherapy of hypertension. Based on recent trials, some general recommendations for the treatment of hypertension in people with diabetes have emerged. ACE inhibitors, ARBs, β-blockers, diuretics, and calcium-channel antagonists have all been shown to reduce cardiovascular events in diabetes. The selection of individual agents depends on the clinical characteristics of the individual, and there are cautions due to diabetes. In particular, elderly patients with diabetes should have their blood pressure lowered gradually, as they can experience significant hypotension on initiation of therapy. Commonly, two or more drugs are needed to adequately control hypertension in this population.

All subjects with diabetes requiring antihypertensive therapy should be treated with a regimen that includes an ACE inhibitor or an ARB. ACE inhibitors and ARBs are attractive choices because they have unique renal protective effects, of particular importance in people with diabetes, and have demonstrated a benefit of reducing cardiovascular disease risk compared to other agents and/or independent of blood pressure–lowering effects. However, some caution is appropriate. Renal insufficiency may worsen in patients with bilateral renal artery stenosis, a problem that may be silent and more common in type 2 diabetes. Diabetic nephropathy is associated with hyporeninemic hypoaldosteronism, and ACE inhibitors and ARBs may cause unacceptable hyperkalemia in these patients. ARBs may be substituted for an ACE inhibitor if unacceptable side effects occur; these agents tend to cause less hyperkalemia and cough.

Table 5.2 Blood Pressure Targets (mmHg) in Individuals with Diabetes

	Systolic	Diastolic
Goal	<130	<80
Behavioral therapy alone (maximum 3 months), then add pharmacologic treatment	130–139	80–89
Behavioral therapy + pharmacologic treatment	≥140	≥90

Based on multiple studies, a thiazide diuretic such as chlorthalidone (25 mg/day) should be used among the first two drugs for managing hypertension in patients with diabetes. The benefit of thiazide diuretics may be particularly large in African-American patients. Rare patients will exhibit significant deterioration in glycemic control, particularly if hypokalemia complicates diuretic therapy. In patients with diabetes and refractory hypertension, more intensive diuresis employing the addition of loop diuretics to reduce intravascular volume can be particularly effective, especially in those with renal insufficiency or evidence of volume overload.

Patients with diabetes and prior MI, angina, or congestive heart failure should be treated with a β-blocker, as these agents have been shown to reduce the risk of death. Treatment with a β-blocker can rarely result in worsening of glycemic control, which can easily be overcome with modification of the diabetes treatment program. β-Blockers have also been suggested to reduce symptoms of hypoglycemia by interfering with adrenergic responses. Patients should be counseled in this regard, but β-blockers should not be withheld in patients with coronary disease or heart failure except potentially in the setting of documented severe hypoglycemia.

Calcium-channel blockers are among the most effective blood pressure–lowering agents. As monotherapy in head-to-head studies, they have generally had more modest effects on cardiovascular disease risk than the other classes listed above. However, verapamil and the dihydropyridine calcium-channel blockers clearly have a place in combination with ACE inhibitors and ARBs in reducing cardiovascular disease events in diabetes.

Central sympatholytic agents may worsen orthostatic hypotension and sexual dysfunction. Peripheral α-blockers as monotherapy have been associated with a higher risk of congestive heart failure than thiazide diuretics and should not be used as first-line therapy in managing hypertension. Caution is necessary when initiating ACE inhibitor therapy in patients on diuretics because hypotension may occur.

Management of Dyslipidemia

In type 2 diabetes, an increased prevalence of lipid abnormalities contributes to accelerated atherosclerosis. Characteristically, triglyceride-rich VLDL levels are elevated, and HDL cholesterol levels, particularly the larger, more beneficial HDL2, are decreased. LDL cholesterol levels are usually not different from those found in age- and sex-matched individuals without diabetes, but the LDL particles may be smaller and more dense, more oxidized, and glycated, all of which increases atherogenicity. Associated obesity aggravates the lipid abnormalities. This lipid profile is the result of a combination of altered synthesis, catabolism, and clearance. A fasting lipid profile is recommended at initial evaluation and at least annually in people with type 2 diabetes. In adults with low-risk lipid values (HDL cholesterol >60 mg/dl, triglyceride <150 mg/dl, and LDL cholesterol <100 mg/dl), repeat assessments can be performed every 2 years.

The Adult Treatment Panel III subcommittee of the National Cholesterol Education Program recommendations for the screening and treatment of dyslipidemias are based predominantly on clinical studies in populations without diabetes. The American Diabetes Association has made some minor modifications to these recommendations specific for people with diabetes because of the high risk of atherosclerosis and the difference in the dyslipidemia commonly found.

- All patients with type 2 diabetes should be screened for dyslipidemia during their initial evaluation by measuring a fasting lipid profile, including triglycerides, total cholesterol, HDL cholesterol, and calculated LDL cholesterol. Triglyceride levels elevated >400 mg/dl, common in individuals with type 2 diabetes, invalidates the calculated LDL cholesterol level. In such cases, direct measurements of LDL are recommended.
- The increased relative risk for cardiovascular disease in both men and women with type 2 diabetes and the common coexisting risk factors (e.g., hypertension) place the entire population with type 2 diabetes in a high-risk category.
- Lifestyle modification with reduction of saturated fat and cholesterol intake, weight loss, increased physical activity, and smoking cessation is very important, particularly in reducing triglycerides and increasing HDL cholesterol.
- Lowering LDL cholesterol to <100 mg/dl is the primary goal of therapy.
- In people with diabetes age >40 years with a total cholesterol >135 mg/dl, statin therapy to achieve an LDL reduction of ~30% regardless of baseline LDL level may be an appropriate target.

Lipid level goals for adults with diabetes are given in Table 5.3. In many cases, elevated triglyceride levels can be satisfactorily lowered by improving glycemic control with nutrition therapy, exercise, oral agents, or insulin. Nutrition recommendations for these patients are outlined in Nutrition (see page 36).

Pharmacotherapy of dyslipidemia. When aggressive diet, exercise, and glucose control fail to control dyslipidemia, the addition of LDL cholesterol–lowering drugs or triglyceride-lowering drugs, depending on the lipid profile, is indicated. Treatment of elevated LDL cholesterol is considered to have first priority, and LDL cholesterol should be lowered to <100 mg/dl. Subgroup analysis of the subjects with diabetes in large trials of the HMG CoA-reductase inhibitors (statins) has shown these agents to be effective in reducing cardiovascular events. Statins

Table 5.3 Lipoprotein Level Goals for Adults with Diabetes

	Lipids
LDL cholesterol	<100 mg/dl (<2.6 mmol/l)
HDL cholesterol	>40 mg/dl (>1.1 mmol/l) for men, >50 mg/dl (>1.3 mmol/l) for women
Triglycerides*	<150 mg/dl (<1.7 mmol/l)

*Current NCEP/ATP III guidelines suggest that in patients with triglycerides ≥200 mg/dl, the "non-HDL cholesterol" (total cholesterol – HDL cholesterol) be utilized. The goal is ≤130 mg/dl.

are also the most effective LDL cholesterol–lowering medications available and have an excellent safety profile. In high doses, some statins also reduce triglycerides significantly. Recent studies using statins suggest that lowering LDL cholesterol to 60–70 mg/dl further benefits people with prior MI, including those with type 2 diabetes, compared with lowering LDL cholesterol to 96 mg/dl. Thus, it appears that very aggressive lowering of LDL cholesterol levels may provide additional benefit to reduce heart disease in high-risk populations. In patients who do not achieve LDL cholesterol targets as a result of statin intolerance or for other reasons, bile-acid sequestrants and cholesterol absorption inhibitors can be used to further reduce LDL cholesterol levels.

Fibrates, particularly fenofibrate, and nicotinic acid can reduce LDL cholesterol levels as well but are primarily used to lower triglyceride and raise HDL cholesterol levels. Fibrates and nicotinic acid are associated with a low-level risk of rhabdomyolysis when combined with statins; this risk seems to be lower with fenofibrate than with gemfibrozil and higher at higher doses of statins. Nicotinic acid at moderate doses (750–2,000 mg/day) has been shown to only modestly increase glucose levels in the setting of diabetes; this can usually be managed by adjusting antihyperglycemic therapy.

Nicotinic acid and fibrates both increase HDL cholesterol and lower triglyceride levels and have been demonstrated to decrease cardiovascular morbidity in clinical trials that excluded or had very few patients with type 2 diabetes. In the VA-HIT study, gemfibrozil treatment was associated with a reduction in cardiovascular events in patients with diabetes, clinical cardiovascular disease, and low HDL cholesterol and near-normal LDL cholesterol levels. Combination therapy employing statins and fibrates or niacin may be necessary to achieve lipid targets, but have not been evaluated in outcomes studies for either event reduction or safety. Triglyceride levels >500 mg/dl are considered a risk factor for pancreatitis and should be aggressively managed. In the presence of dyslipidemia characterized predominantly by elevated triglyceride, a fibrate is recommended, but additional therapy with nicotinic acid and ω-3 fatty acids may be required.

Smoking Cessation

Cigarette smoking is associated with accelerated macrovascular disease, and the presence of diabetes in a patient who smokes will further increase that individual's risk. Ongoing efforts should be made by the practitioner to assist the patient in discontinuing cigarette smoking, including enrollment in formal smoking cessation programs, behavioral modification, and use of nicotine patches. Some individuals may benefit from a trial of bupropion HCl to relieve some withdrawal symptoms.

TREATMENT OF CARDIOVASCULAR DISEASE

Clinical trials that examined the efficacy of secondary interventions (after clinical disease has occurred) have often excluded patients with diabetes. However, clinical experience and a limited number of trials in type 2 diabetes suggest similar efficacy of medical and surgical treatments of cardiac, cerebral, and peripheral arterial disease as those in nondiabetic populations, with several caveats. Anti-anginal treatment regimens and treatment of other risk factors after an MI probably provide a similar benefit to both people with and people without diabetes. Clinical trials such as the Norwegian timolol study have included a sufficient number of patients with type 2 diabetes to demonstrate efficacy of β-blockade in preventing a second MI. In insulin- or sulfonylurea-treated patients, the heightened risks of hypoglycemia with β-blockade must be taken into account.

Despite the generally more diffuse coronary and peripheral artery disease in patients with type 2 diabetes compared to patients without diabetes, bypass surgery is an effective treatment, although patients with diabetes do have increased morbidity and mortality. The Bypass Angioplasty Revascularization Investigation found that patients with multiple vessel disease had much better survival when randomized to coronary artery bypass grafting, including internal mammary artery grafting, than did patients undergoing angioplasty. It is not known whether the superiority of surgical approaches will also apply to patients with more focal disease or whether the use of newer stents and glycoprotein IIa/IIIb inhibitors during percutaneous intervention during angioplasty will minimize the differences in outcomes between the two approaches. Studies suggest that glycemic control before and during interventional coronary vessel procedures improves overall patient outcomes.

DIABETIC RETINOPATHY

The importance of frequent evaluation of and early detection and treatment of vision problems in patients with diabetes is illustrated by the following points:

- ~5,000 new cases of blindness related to diabetes are estimated to occur every year in the U.S., making diabetes a leading cause of new blindness among adults age 20–74 years.
- >60% of patients with type 2 diabetes have some degree of retinopathy 20 years after diagnosis. At the same point, nearly all patients with type 1 diabetes have retinopathy.
- Up to 21% of patients with type 2 diabetes have retinopathy at diagnosis.
- Loss of vision associated with proliferative retinopathy and macular edema can be reduced by 50% with laser photocoagulation, if identified in a timely manner.
- Aspirin therapy does not prevent retinopathy or increase the risk of hemorrhage.

As in type 1 diabetes, the development and progression of retinopathy in type 2 diabetes is duration dependent and associated with higher glycemic levels. Keeping glycemia in the near-normal range definitely prevents or delays the onset of retinopathy. High blood pressure is a risk factor for the development of macular edema and is associated with the presence of proliferative retinopathy. Lowering blood pressure decreases the progression of retinopathy. Attempts to normalize glucose and blood pressure levels, especially with low-risk treatments such as nutrition therapy and exercise, are appropriate. Although relatively fewer people with type 2 diabetes versus type 1 diabetes develop proliferative retinopathy, macular edema may

Table 5.4 What Patients Need to Know—Retinopathy

- Inform newly diagnosed patients that vision loss is a possibility and that they must report visual symptoms promptly.
- Instruct patients regarding the relationship between hyperglycemia, hypertension, and diabetic retinopathy, focusing on risk factor control to preserve eyesight.
- Inform patients of the importance of an annual dilated eye examination by an ophthalmologist or optometrist, because retinopathy can develop without symptoms and worsen quickly.
- Reassure patients concerning transient vision changes associated with casual glycemic fluctuations and temporary changes in retinopathy status due to changes in glycemic therapy or pregnancy.
- Inform patients of the sight-saving procedures, including photocoagulation, available for severe nonproliferative and proliferative retinopathy and macular edema.
- Inform patients that isometric exercises that raise intraocular pressure can aggravate proliferative retinopathy.
- Suggest support programs and community services for patients with visual impairments or blindness.

be more common. In addition to retinopathy, patients with type 2 diabetes develop cataracts more frequently and at an earlier age than do people without diabetes.

Diabetic retinopathy does not cause visual symptoms until at a fairly advanced stage, usually when either proliferative retinopathy or macular edema is present. Management is more satisfactory when intervention is undertaken before visual symptoms develop. Therefore, yearly ophthalmoscopic examination by an ophthalmologist or optometrist who is experienced in diagnosing diabetic retinopathy is of crucial importance.

The frequency of visual impairment related to diabetes makes effective patient education crucial. Table 5.4 presents patient teaching points concerning retinopathy.

STAGES OF DIABETIC RETINOPATHY

Nonproliferative Diabetic Retinopathy

Nonproliferative diabetic retinopathy is the earliest stage and is characterized by microaneurysms and intraretinal "dot and blot" hemorrhages. Most individuals with long-term type 2 diabetes eventually develop it, but in many cases, it does not progress and has no effect on visual acuity. However, if the abnormal vessels leak serous fluid in the area of the maculae, which is responsible for central vision, macular edema can occur with disruption of the usual transmission of light and result in a decrease in visual acuity. Macular edema may be mild and not immediately threaten vision or may be clinically significant macular edema and require treatment because of the immediate threat to central vision. The presence of macular edema is suspected if there are hard exudates in close proximity to the maculae. Circinate hard exudates near the maculae are especially suspicious. Any of these findings should prompt referral to an ophthalmologist or optometrist with expertise in diabetic retinopathy.

Severe Nonproliferative Retinopathy

Certain retinal lesions represent an advanced form of nonproliferative retinopathy. These lesions include cotton-wool spots (also referred to as soft exudates), which are ischemic infarcts in the inner retinal layers; "beading" of the retinal veins; and intraretinal microvascular abnormalities, which are dilated, tortuous retinal capillaries or, perhaps in some cases, newly formed vessels within the retina. When these lesions are found together, the risk of progression to the proliferative stage is increased, and presence of any of these signs should prompt referral to an ophthalmologist or optometrist who is knowledgeable and experienced in the management of diabetic retinopathy without delay.

Proliferative Diabetic Retinopathy

The most vision-threatening stage of diabetic retinopathy is characterized by neovascularization on the surface of the retina, sometimes extending into the posterior vitreous. These vessels probably develop in response to ischemia. The prevalence of proliferative retinopathy among people who have had type 2 diabetes for >20 years may approach 30%. Proliferative retinopathy threatens vision because the new vessels are prone to bleed, especially if they are stretched by contraction of the vitreous. If bleeding into the preretinal space or vitreous occurs, the patient is likely to report "floaters" or "cobwebs" in the field of vision. The patient who has a major retinal hemorrhage will experience a sudden, painless loss of vision. The proliferation of fibrous tissue that often follows can lead to retinal detachment as fibrous tissue contracts.

PREVENTION OF RETINOPATHY

Both the Diabetes Control and Complications Trial (DCCT) and the UKPDS demonstrated that intensive treatment that lowers average glucose levels to near normal prevents or ameliorates retinopathy. Additionally, the small Kumamoto study in Japan demonstrated benefit of improved control in type 2 patients, and the Wisconsin Epidemiologic Study of Diabetic Retinopathy found a strong association between baseline glycated hemoglobin and progression of retinopathy in type 2 patients independent of treatment. Also, two large prospective studies, the Diabetic Retinopathy Study and the Early Treatment of Diabetic Retinopathy Study, provided strong support for the benefits of photocoagulation therapy, which decreases loss of vision in patients with proliferative retinopathy or macular edema. Therefore, identification of patients at risk in a timely manner is a major means of preventing loss of vision. The UKPDS also provided evidence that blood pressure control prevents the appearance and progression of retinopathy.

Evaluation and Referral

The changes involved in diabetic retinopathy may be subtle and escape detection by direct ophthalmoscopy. All patients with type 2 diabetes should have an annual examination with complete visual history, visual acuity examination, and

Table 5.5 Indications for Referral of Patients with Type 2 Diabetes Mellitus to an Ophthalmologist or Optometrist

■ High-risk patients—immediate referral
  • Neovascularization covering more than 1/3 of optic disk
  • Vitreous or preretinal hemorrhage with any neovascularization, particularly on optic disk
  • Macular edema
■ Symptomatic patients
  • Blurry vision persisting for >1–2 days not associated with change in blood glucose
  • Sudden loss of vision in one or both eyes
  • Black spots, cobwebs, or flashing lights in field of vision
■ Asymptomatic patients
  • Annual examinations
  • Hard exudates near macula
  • Any preproliferative or proliferative characteristics
  • Pregnancy

careful ophthalmoscopic examination with a dilated pupil by an ophthalmologist or optometrist. The annual evaluations should begin at diagnosis of type 2 diabetes, because the duration of hyperglycemia before diagnosis is uncertain and many patients have established retinopathy at diagnosis. The indications for referral are listed in Table 5.5. Nondilated photographic retinal screening is available, but it is not considered a replacement for the annual examination because no rigorous studies have demonstrated equivalent diagnostic accuracy.

Note that visual acuity changes are frequently related to fluctuating glycemic levels and corresponding changes in hydration of the crystalline lens. Thus, a presenting symptom of diabetes in a patient may be a change in vision. Likewise, a patient whose glycemic levels are decreased in response to proper treatment may experience visual acuity changes and should be forewarned as well as reassured.

TREATMENT OF RETINOPATHY

The ophthalmologic treatment of diabetic retinopathy depends on the stage of disease. There is no commonly accepted therapy for nonproliferative retinopathy other than improved glycemic and blood pressure control. Panretinal photocoagulation is considered the treatment of choice for patients who have proliferative retinopathy with high-risk characteristics, and it reduces the risk of severe visual loss by about 60%. Photocoagulation slows progressive visual loss in patients with macular edema by 50%.

Photocoagulation is used to stop neovascularization before recurrent hemorrhages into the vitreous cause irreparable damage. Sometimes photocoagulation is used to treat eyes with proliferative retinopathy before high-risk characteristics have developed. However, the risks of photocoagulation are such that usually only one eye is treated; treatment of the other eye is deferred unless high-risk characteristics develop. If retinal detachment and massive vitreous hemorrhage occur, closed vitrectomy can be used to remove bloody vitreous and bands of fibrous tissue. During the procedure, clear fluid is infused to replace vitreous, and traction on the retina is relieved. In ~50–65% of cases, some sight can be restored with this procedure.

DIABETIC RENAL DISEASE

Diabetic nephropathy occurs in 20–40% of individuals with diabetes and is the leading cause of end-stage renal disease (ESRD). More than 40% of new cases of ESRD, >40,000 annually, are due to diabetes. The incidence of ESRD is four times higher in African Americans, four to six times higher in Mexican Americans, and six times higher in Native Americans than in the general population of those with diabetes. The frequency of kidney disease related to diabetes makes effective patient education crucial. Table 5.6 presents patient teaching points concerning nephropathy.

CLINICAL PRESENTATION OF NEPHROPATHY

The development of diabetic nephropathy is asymptomatic, and its detection relies on laboratory screening. The usual course of diabetic nephropathy in type 2 diabetes is not as stereotypical as in type 1 diabetes, but nephropathy tends to progress through several defined stages. The first sign of developing nephropathy is the occurrence of elevated microalbuminuria (>30 mg albumin/24 h). Whether microalbuminuria carries the same risk for the eventual development of clinical nephropathy in type 2 diabetes, as seems to be the case in type 1 diabetes, is unclear. As nephropathy progresses, "clinical" (dipstick positive, >300 mg albuminuria/24 h) proteinuria occurs, almost always concurrent with hypertension. Eventually, nephrotic-range proteinuria develops, followed by decreasing glomerular filtration rate with rising serum creatinine, until ESRD occurs.

Table 5.6 What Patients Need to Know—Nephropathy

- Optimizing glycemic control prevents or delays nephropathy.
- Annual urine tests are the only way to detect the "silent" onset of diabetic kidney disease.
- Regular blood pressure checks are vital because untreated hypertension damages the kidney, precipitates the onset of renal disease, and accelerates its progression.
- Effectively treating hypertension, with medication, weight loss, and/or sodium restriction, will help prevent or slow the progression of diabetic kidney disease.
- People with diabetes have an increased risk for urinary tract infections. Inform patients of the symptoms they need to detect and report.
- If there are signs of developing nephropathy, explain the course of the disease and the options for treatment with dialysis and renal transplantation.

CONDITIONS THAT INFLUENCE RENAL FUNCTION

In patients with diabetes, several conditions either precipitate the development of nephropathy or exacerbate the condition when present.

- **Hypertension** may precipitate the onset or further accelerate the process of renal insufficiency, or both. Virtually all patients with diabetes who develop nephropathy develop hypertension.
- **Neurogenic bladder** may predispose the patient to acute urinary retention or to moderate and persistent obstructive nephropathy. In either case, renal failure may be accelerated.
- When **infection and urinary obstruction** occur together, the risk of pyelonephritis and papillary necrosis increases, and this may result in a decline of renal function. Repetitive urethral instrumentation increases the risk of urinary tract infections. Infarction of the renal medulla and papillae can occur from ischemic necrosis and infarction or obstruction and is typically accompanied by fever, flank pain, anuria, and accelerated loss of renal function.
- **Nephrotoxic drugs,** such as nonsteroidal anti-inflammatory drugs, chronic analgesic abuse, and contrast media used in radiographic studies, have been associated with increased incidence and acceleration of renal failure in patients with diabetes. Nephrotoxic drugs should be avoided, and contrast media studies should be performed only after careful consideration of alternative procedures and with adequate hydration.

PREVENTION AND TREATMENT OF DIABETIC RENAL DISEASE

As with retinopathy, the DCCT and UKPDS demonstrated a decrease in development of microalbuminuria and clinical grade proteinuria with improved metabolic control. The UKPDS also showed that control of blood pressure reduces the risk for the development of nephropathy.

Three methods can be utilized for microalbuminuria screening: measurement of the albumin-to-creatinine ratio in a random spot collection; 24-h collection with creatinine, allowing the simultaneous measurement of creatinine clearance; or a timed (e.g., 4-h or overnight) collection. The spot measurement of the albumin-to-creatinine ratio is the easiest to perform and has a good predictive value. A value of >30 mg/g creatinine is considered abnormal. There is a diurnal variation, and the spot urine should be done in the morning if possible. A value >30 mg/24 h is considered abnormal as is a value >20 µg/min in a timed specimen. In addition to screening for microalbuminuria, a urinalysis (including microscopic analysis) and serum creatinine should be done in all newly diagnosed patients.

The finding of increased microalbuminuria or proteinuria should be followed by measurement of serum creatinine or urea nitrogen concentrations and assessment of glomerular filtration. If present, infection should be treated before the significance of the proteinuria can be determined. Consultation with a specialist is suggested if persistent proteinuria, an elevation in serum creatinine, a glomerular filtration rate <60 ml/min, or hypertension unresponsive to treatment is seen.

The presence of microalbuminuria may be the first indication of advancing nephropathy and, if present, should prompt aggressive treatment of even modestly elevated blood pressure. To delay the onset and acceleration of renal disease in patients with diabetes, hypertension must be detected and treated aggressively. The ACE inhibitors and ARBs are particularly beneficial in this regard. In type 1 diabetes, ACE inhibitors have been shown to slow the progression for micro- to macroalbuminuria and the decline in glomerular filtration rate. In subjects with type 2 diabetes, ARBs have also been shown to reduce the risk of progression from micro- to macroalbuminuria as well as ESRD. Dihydroperidine calcium-channel blockers should only be utilized to achieve blood pressure targets in patients already treated with an ACE inhibitor or ARB. There are potential complications associated with the use of antihypertensive medications to be kept in mind when instituting therapy (see Pharmacotherapy of hypertension, page 104).

DIABETIC FOOT PROBLEMS

More than 50% of the nontraumatic amputations in the U.S. occur in individuals with diabetes, and it has been estimated that >50% of these amputations could have been prevented with proper care. Therefore, the clinician and patient who are conscientious about prevention, early detection, and prompt treatment of diabetic foot problems can make a significant impact on this complication.

CAUSES OF FOOT PROBLEMS

Foot lesions in individuals with diabetes mellitus are the result of polyneuropathy, peripheral arterial disease, superimposed infection, or, most often, a combination of these complications. Usually, foot lesions begin in feet that are insensitive, deformed, and/or ischemic. Such feet are susceptible to trauma, which may lead to callus formation, ulceration, infection, and gangrene.

In most patients with diabetes who have foot lesions, the primary pathophysiologic event is the development of an insensitive foot secondary to polyneuropathy. Loss of foot sensation is often, but not always, accompanied by decreased vibratory sense and loss of ankle deep tendon reflexes. Sometimes, diabetic neuropathy is accompanied and worsened by other types of neuropathy, most commonly alcoholic or uremic peripheral neuropathy.

In addition to insensitivity, neuropathy may ultimately lead to a deformed foot secondary to tendon shortening (contractures), which leads to decreased mobility of the toes, abnormality in weight bearing, calluses, and development of classic "hammer toe" deformities. The combination of foot insensitivity and foot deformities that shift weight distribution promotes the development of foot ulcers. Neuropathy also causes decreased sweating and dry skin. If left untreated, cracked and thickened skin can lead to infections and ulcerations. Neuropathic ulcers in the patient with diabetes often go undetected because they are usually painless.

Neuroarthropathy (Charcot arthropathy) is an underrecognized complication of diabetic neuropathy that can result in disabling foot deformities. It usually occurs in the presence of adequate circulation. It is characterized by disintegration and disorganization of the bones in the lower leg and foot and can be precipitated by minimal trauma. Early recognition and appropriate treatment can substantially reduce permanent deformities.

The sudden development of a painful distal foot lesion, usually secondary to trauma, may signify underlying peripheral arterial disease, which is associated with findings of decreased or absent pulses, dependent rubor, and pallor on elevation. The extent of the vascular disease and its potential for treatment by surgical intervention can be determined by Doppler noninvasive techniques and arteriography. Revascularization procedures, such as angioplasty and bypass, are often helpful in treating patients with severe, disabling claudication (at rest) or nonhealing ulcers or to aid healing of an amputation incision. Unfortunately, surgical intervention is not always effective in individuals with diabetes because many have diffuse vascular disease.

Infection is a frequent complication of both vascular and neuropathic ulcers. Studies indicate that these infections are often mixed and that gram-positive organisms predominate.

PREVENTION OF FOOT PROBLEMS

The prevention of foot problems in a person with diabetes requires proper foot care by the patient as well as early detection and prompt treatment of lesions by the physician. Help from health care specialists, e.g., podiatrist, orthopedist, vascular surgeon, expert shoe fitter, is frequently needed.

The first step in prevention is to educate all patients and to identify those who need specialized or frequent evaluations because of risk factors for foot problems (Table 5.7). During the evaluation, the examiner should determine whether the patient has experienced foot problems or intermittent claudication since the last visit. The physician also should conduct a thorough examination of both feet, looking for the signs and symptoms of impending foot problems (Table 5.8), including foot deformities, calluses, and ulcers. The clinician should also check the pulses (dorsalis pedis, posterior tibial, and femoral), search for bruits, and determine reflexes and sensation in the toes and feet. Evaluation of neurologic status in the foot should involve the use of the Semmes-Weinstein 5.07 (10-g) monofilament (Table 5.9; Fig. 5.1).

Table 5.7 What Patients Need to Know—Foot Care

- The patient, or family member in the case of a patient who is impaired by morbid obesity or blindness, has the major responsibility for prevention of foot problems.
- Cut toenails straight across and inspect the feet daily for cuts, abrasions, and corns.
- Regular washing with warm water and mild soap followed by thorough drying is essential.
- Use moistening agents, such as lanolin, as needed.
- Avoid prolonged soaking, strong chemicals such as Epsom salts or iodine, and "home surgery."
- Heat, cold, new shoes, constricting or mended socks, and, perhaps most important, going barefoot are potential hazards that must be emphasized to all patients, especially those with peripheral neuropathy.

Table 5.8 Warning Symptoms and Signs of Diabetic Foot Problems

	Symptoms	Signs
Vascular	Cold feet Intermittent claudication involving calf or foot Pain at rest, especially nocturnal, relieved by dependency	Absent pedal, popliteal, or femoral pulses Femoral bruits Dependent rubor, plantar pallor on elevation Prolonged capillary filling time (>3–4 s) Decreased skin temperature
Neurologic	Sensory: burning, tingling, or crawling sensations; pain and hypersensitivity, cold feet Hand symptoms Motor: weakness (foot drop) Autonomic: diminished sweating	Sensory: deficits (vibratory, light touch and proprioceptive, pain and temperature perception), hyperesthesia Carpal tunnel syndrome (paresthesiae, sensory loss over median distribution) Motor: diminished to absent deep tendon reflexes (Achilles, then patellar), weakness, wasting Autonomic: diminished to absent sweating Heat and edema due to increased arteriovenous shunting
Musculoskeletal	Gradual change in foot shape, sudden painless change in foot shape, with swelling, without history or trauma Weakness of hand muscles	Cavus feet with claw toes Drop foot "Rocker-bottom" foot Neuropathic arthropathy (Charcot's joint) Wasting
Dermatologic	Exquisitely painful or painless wounds Slow-healing or nonhealing wounds or necrosis Skin color changes (cyanosis, redness) Chronic scaling, itching or dry feet Recurrent infections (e.g., paronychia, athlete's foot)	Skin: abnormal dryness Chronic tinea infections Keratotic lesions with or without hemorrhage (plantar or digital) Trophic ulcer Hair: diminished or absent Nails: trophic changes Onychomycosis Sublingual ulceration or abscess Ingrown nails with paronychia

Table 5.9 Physician-Performed Monofilament Examination

- Examination must be done in a quiet and relaxed supine patient's with position, with closed eyes.
- First, apply the monofilament on the patient's hands to teach him or her what to feel. The patient must not be able to see whether the filament is being applied.
- Three sites are tested on each foot: the big toe pulp and the 1st and 5th metatarsus heads.
- Apply the filament perpendicular to test skin surface with sufficient force to cause the filament to bend ~45°; the entire procedure should take ~2 s.
- Ask the patient *if* and *where* he or she felt pressure applied.
- Repeat the measurement twice at each site per foot in random order.
- Express the result separately for each foot in a ratio, e.g., 4/6 means the patient felt 4 touches of 6, 6/6 means the patient felt each application.
- During the procedure, test twice by a blind application the patient's drive to comply with you. If the patient answers positively while no filament is applied, cancel everything, further explain this procedure and its importance, and repeat entire procedure.

TREATMENT OF FOOT PROBLEMS

Minor noninfected wounds can be treated with nonirritating antiseptic solution, daily dressing changes, and foot rest. More serious problems, such as foot deformities, infected lesions, and osteomyelitis, are best handled in consultation with specialists in diabetic foot care. Infected foot ulcers usually require intravenous antibiotics, bed rest with foot elevation, and surgical debridement. Reducing plantar pressure using contact casts/specialized footware accelerates healing.

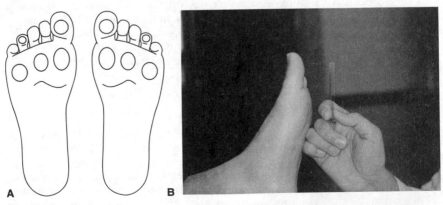

A   B

Figure 5.1 Sites (*A*) for Semmes-Weinstein monofilament testing (*B*).

NEUROPATHIC CONDITIONS

The diabetic neuropathies are among the most common and perplexing complications of diabetes mellitus. Neuropathy has a wide variety of manifestations in people with diabetes, and the descriptive terminology and classification have also varied, causing some confusion among clinicians. A complete dissertation on neuropathy is beyond the scope of this book section. Instead, a few important points about diagnosis and treatment of commonly encountered neuropathic problems are discussed.

POLYNEUROPATHY

Polyneuropathy begins as a generalized, asymptomatic dysfunction of sensorimotor or autonomic peripheral nerve fibers. The sensorimotor neuropathy is symmetric and first involves the distal lower extremities. The presence and severity of the neuropathy generally relates to the duration of diabetes and degree of hyperglycemia. In people with type 2 diabetes, polyneuropathy may be present at diagnosis. Painful neuropathy has been identified in subjects with pre-diabetes. Polyneuropathy is often associated with retinopathy and nephropathy.

Several stages in the progression of polyneuropathy have been identified. The first abnormality is an asymptomatic change in nerve conduction or reduction of the heartbeat response to deep breathing or the Valsalva maneuver. To define neuropathy, the changes should be present in two or more nerves. Next, the patient is found to have decreased or absent ankle reflexes and/or abnormal vibratory sensation of the great toes. When present, symptoms can be either pain or relate to a loss of function. The pain intensity varies from causing discomfort to being disabling and may be described as sticking, lancinating, prickling, burning, aching, boring, and/or excessively sensitive. Fortunately, most patients do not have pain, and when present, the pain may be a transitory phase.

Loss of pain does not necessarily imply improvement in the neuropathy. Functional loss is more common and is manifested by decreased tactile sense, lack of temperature discrimination, sensory loss, and muscle weakness. Inability to walk on the heels is a sign of more severe neuropathy. The muscular weakness may lead to foot deformity, such as hammertoes and abnormal weight bearing. The insensitivity leads to neglect of injury and contributes to foot ulcers (neurotrophic ulcers) and Charcot's joint. Although polyneuropathy can affect the hands, most often, hand symptoms are caused by carpal tunnel syndrome or ulnar neuropathy.

AUTONOMIC NEUROPATHY

Diminished autonomic nerve function can cause an interesting variety of symptoms. Autonomic polyneuropathy, which usually occurs in concert with peripheral sensorimotor neuropathy, includes gastroparesis, diabetic diarrhea, constipation, neurogenic bladder, gustatory sweating, impaired cardiovascular reflexes and orthostatic hypotension, sexual dysfunction in men, and dyspareunia in women. Clinically, autonomic neuropathy tends to appear late in the course of diabetes.

Gastroparesis

Severe, symptomatic gastroparesis is uncommon in people with type 2 diabetes. However, when present, the patient with gastroparesis may experience early satiety, nausea, vomiting, abdominal discomfort, and fluctuations of postprandial blood glucose levels secondary to delayed emptying or retention of gastric contents. Other upper gastrointestinal abnormalities must be excluded before making a diagnosis of gastroparesis. Gastric emptying studies may be necessary to confirm the diagnosis, but may not correlate with symptoms. However, significant hyperglycemia can temporarily delay gastric emptying, so glycemic control during the test should be monitored. Metoclopramide is often helpful in treating gastroparesis. Erythromycin and nortriptyline have been shown to improve gastric emptying and benefit some patients. Domperidone is an investigational drug that has been shown to be effective (available in Canada).

Diabetic Diarrhea

Frequent passage of loose stools, particularly after meals and at night, marks the acute phase of this condition. Diabetic diarrhea tends to be intermittent and may alternate with constipation. Diphenoxylate, loperamide, and clonidine have been shown to be effective to some degree. Some patients respond to treatment with a broad-spectrum antibiotic such as tetracycline. In resistant cases, parenteral octreotide can be helpful.

Neurogenic Bladder

Neurogenic bladder is characterized by a pattern of frequent, small voidings and incontinence and may progress to urinary retention. The demonstration of cystometric abnormalities and large residual urine volume are necessary for diagnosis. The patient with significant urinary retention may need to perform intermittent self-catheterization. Surgical intervention may rarely be required if the patient does not respond to conservative medical measures, because chronic urinary retention may lead to infection.

Impaired Cardiovascular Reflexes

Orthostatic hypotension and increased heart rate may occur when autonomic neuropathy affects the cardiovascular reflexes. Patients with orthostatic hypotension may require adjustment of concurrent aggravating medications and may find relief by elevating the head of the bed and with the use of fludrocortisone and compression stockings. If fludrocortisone is prescribed, the initial dose should be 0.1 mg/day, and increases up to 0.4 mg/day should be made gradually. The drug should be used with particular caution in patients with cardiac disease, because it causes sodium and water retention and thus can precipitate congestive heart failure. Clonidine, a central $\alpha2$-receptor–blocking agent, has been used to treat this condition. Midodine is a newer agent that has been shown to benefit some patients.

Sexual Dysfunction in Men

Sexual dysfunction is a frequent occurrence in men with diabetes and usually manifests as lack of a firm, sustained erection. In most cases, libido and ejaculatory function are not affected, although retrograde ejaculation may be another feature of autonomic neuropathy. The measurement of nocturnal penile tumescence is sometimes used to determine whether the patient's erections during sleep are normal, borderline, or abnormally diminished for age. When psychological and endocrine causes of impotence have been ruled out, the use of 5' phosphodiesterase inhibitors (i.e., sildanafil, vardenafil, tadalafil), vacuum devices, intrapenile injections of vasodilating substances (e.g., papaverine, phentolamine, prostaglandin), or intraurethral insertion of medication (alprostadil) allow the patient to resume sexual intercourse. The implantation of an inflatable or semirigid prosthesis is usually not required in the older patient with type 2 diabetes.

OTHER VARIETIES OF DIABETIC NEUROPATHY

In addition to symmetric polyneuropathy, people with diabetes are subject to a variety of other neuropathic syndromes. These syndromes include lumbosacral plexus neuropathies (also called femoral neuropathy or diabetic amyotrophy), truncal radiculopathy, upper limb mononeuropathies (the entrapment neuropathies—carpal tunnel syndrome and ulnar neuropathy, which are more common in people with diabetes), and cranial neuropathy. These varieties of neuropathy are asymmetric and abrupt or subacute in onset and tend to follow a monophasic course with improvement over time. They may be more common in type 2 diabetes, and their association with hyperglycemia is less clear-cut than that of polyneuropathy. In some cases, there is evidence that ischemia or inflammation is involved. Patients have more than one type of diabetic neuropathy.

Lumbosacral plexus neuropathy may present with abrupt onset of asymmetric lower limb proximal muscle pain and weakness or, in its most severe form, with severe pain, wasting of the proximal muscles, and modest sensory involvement (diabetic amyotrophy). It is more common in men with type 2 diabetes. Prominent features include quadriceps involvement, atrophy of thigh muscles, and absent patellar tendon reflexes. Recovery usually occurs in several months to a year. However, the condition may recur contralaterally.

Extraocular muscle motor paralysis, particularly that innervated by the third and sixth nerves, is the most noticeable of the cranial mononeuropathies. Patients can also develop peroneal (foot drop) and median or ulnar palsies. Spontaneous recovery in about 3–6 months is usual.

DIAGNOSIS AND TREATMENT OF NEUROPATHY

The diagnosis of diabetic neuropathy is often easily made on clinical evaluation with little testing necessary. People with diabetes can have neuropathy unrelated to their diabetes. When the clinical features are not typical (i.e., unilateral, predominantly upper limb, rapidly progressive, mainly motor) or consistent with the duration of diabetes and presence of other complications, other causes of neuropathy should be excluded.

There is little evidence that any drug therapy is useful in preventing or curing diabetic neuropathy. Treatment with tricyclic antidepressant medication such as nortriptyline, or antiseizure medications such as gabapentin, lamictal, or carbamazepine may be helpful in some patients with painful neuropathy. Other successful treatments include tramadol and lidoderm patches. A topical cream, capsaicin, is variably effective. Aspirin, propoxyphene, and other analgesics should be prescribed as necessary for pain. Narcotics have reduced efficacy and, in general, should be withheld until all other treatment modalities have been exhausted. Physical therapy methods of treatment are often helpful. Referral to a pain clinic may be necessary.

BIBLIOGRAPHY

Adler AI, Stratton IM, Neil HA, Yudkin JS, Mathews DR, Cull CA, Wright AD, Turner RC, Holman RR: Association of systolic blood pressure with macrovascular and microvascular complications of type 2 diabetes (UKPDS 36): prospective observational study. *BMJ* 321:412–419, 2000

American Diabetes Association: Aspirin therapy in diabetes (Position Statement). *Diabetes Care* 27 (Suppl. 1):S72–S73, 2004

American Diabetes Association: Consensus development conference on the diagnosis of coronary heart disease in people with diabetes (Consensus Statement). *Diabetes Care* 21:1551–1559, 1998

American Diabetes Association: Preventive foot care in diabetes (Position Statement). *Diabetes Care* 27 (Suppl. 1):S63–S64, 2004

Arauz-Pacheco C, Parrott MA, Raskin P: The treatment of hypertension in adult patients with diabetes mellitus (Technical Review). *Diabetes Care* 25:134–147, 2002

Bakris GL, Williams M, Dworkin L, Elliot WJ, Epstein M, Toto R, Tuttle K, Douglas J, Hsueh W, Sowers J: Preserving renal function in adults with hypertension and diabetes: a consensus approach. *Am J Kidney Dis* 36:646–661, 2000

BARI Investigators: Influence of diabetes on 5-year mortality and morbidity in a randomized trial comparing CABG and PTCA in patients with multivessel disease. *Circulation* 96:1761–1769, 1997

Brenner BM, Cooper ME, de Zeeuw D, Keane WF, Mitch WE, Parving HH, Remuzzi G, Snapinn SM, Zhang Z, Shahinfar S: Effects of losartan on renal and cardiovascular outcomes in patients with nephropathy due to type 2 diabetes. *N Engl J Med* 345:861–869, 2001

Chobanian AV, Bakris GL, Black HR, Cushman WC, Green LA, Izzo JL Jr, Jones DW, Materson BJ, Oparil S, Wright JT Jr, Roccella EJ, the National Heart, Lung, and Blood Institute Joint National Committee on Prevention, Detection, Evaluation, and Treatment of High Blood Pressure, the National High Blood Pressure Education Program Coordinating Committee: The Seventh Report of the Joint National Committee on Prevention, Detection, Evaluation, and Treatment of High Blood Pressure: the JNC 7 report. *JAMA* 289:2560–2572, 2003

DCCT/EDIC Research Group: Retinopathy and nephropathy in patients with type 1 diabetes four years after a trial of intensive therapy. *N Engl J Med* 342:381–389, 2000

DCCT Research Group: The effect of intensive diabetes therapy on the development and progression of neuropathy. *Ann Intern Med* 122:561–568, 1995

DCCT Research Group: The effect of intensive treatment of diabetes on the development and progression of long-term complications in insulin-dependent diabetes mellitus. *N Engl J Med* 329:977–986, 1993

Feldman EL, Stevens MJ, Russell JW, Greene DA: Somatosensory neuropathy. In *Ellenberg and Rifkin's Diabetes Mellitus.* Porte D Jr, Sherwin RS, Baron A, Eds. New York, McGraw Hill, 2002, p. 771–788

Hansson L, Zanchetti A, Carruthers SG, Dahlof B, Elmfield D, Julius S, Manard J, Rahn KH, Wedel H, Westerling S: Effects of intensive blood-pressure lowering and low-dose aspirin on patients with hypertension: principal results of the Hypertension Optimal Treatment (HOT) random-ized trial: HOT Study Group. *Lancet* 351:1755–1762, 1998

Heart Outcomes Prevention Evaluation (HOPE) Study Investigators: Effects of ramipril on cardiovascular outcomes in people with diabetes mellitus: results of the HOPE study and MICRO-HOPE study. *Lancet* 355:253–259, 2000

Heart Protection Study Collaborative Group: MRC/BHF Heart Protection Study of cholesterol-lowering with simvastatin in 5963 people with diabetes: a randomized placebo-controlled trial. *Lancet* 361:2005–2016, 2003

National Cholesterol Education Program (NCEP) Expert Panel on Detection, Evaluation, and Treatment of High Blood Cholesterol in Adults (Adult Treatment Panel III): Executive summary of the third report of the National Cholesterol Education Program (NCEP) Expert Panel on the Detection, Evaluation, and Treatment of High Blood Cholesterol in Adults (Adult Treatment Panel III). *JAMA* 285:2486–2497, 2001

Ohkubo Y, Kishikawa H, Araki E, Isami S, Motoyoshi S, Kojima Y, Furuyoshi N, Shichiri M: Intensive insulin therapy prevents the progression of diabetic microvascular complications in Japanese patients with non-insulin-dependent diabetes mellitus: a randomized prospective 6-year study. *Diabetes Res Clin Pract* 28:103–117, 1995

UK Prospective Diabetes Study (UKPDS) Group: Effect of intensive blood-glucose control with metformin on complications in overweight patients with type 2 diabetes (UKPDS 34). *Lancet* 352:854–865, 1998

UK Prospective Diabetes Study (UKPDS) Group: Intensive blood-glucose control with sulphonylureas or insulin compared with conventional treatment and risk of complications in patients with type 2 diabetes (UKPDS 33). *Lancet* 352:837–853, 1998

UK Prospective Diabetes Study (UKPDS) Group: Tight blood pressure control and risk of macrovascular and microvascular complications of type 2 diabetes (UKPDS 38). *BMJ* 317:703–713, 1998

Behavior Change in Diabetes

Highlights

Influences on Behavior Change

Strategies for Behavior Change

Self-Management Support

Redesigning Practice to Support Behavior Change

Conclusion

Highlights
Behavior Change
in Diabetes

■ Most diabetes care is actually self-care that requires patients to actively participate in decision-making, goal-setting, and the process of daily management.

■ Multiple behavioral changes are often required for patients to manage diabetes effectively and achieve their desired level of glycemic control. Making and sustaining the behavioral changes needed for diabetes self-management requires collaboration between the patient and provider to develop a relevant, useful plan.

■ To succeed, patients need diabetes education followed by ongoing self-management and psychosocial support. Involving the entire health care team in this process increases the likelihood of success.

Behavior Change in Diabetes

Diabetes requires considerable effort on the part of patients, regardless of the treatment approach. Patients are often asked to adjust eating patterns and selection of foods, increase their activity, monitor blood glucose levels, take multiple medications, lose weight, perform foot care, and make multiple decisions each day based on blood glucose levels, activity, and food choices. In addition to these behavioral changes, patients need to cope with the stresses and emotional impact of knowing they have a chronic illness that can result in multiple complications and premature death. Although the use of more intensive regimens offers greater hope for a healthier future, these regimens also increase the complexity and demands for self-care and behavior change. Regardless of the type of treatment program, the patient is ultimately responsible for its implementation.

This responsibility for behavior change and self-care is based on three characteristics of diabetes—choices, control, and consequences. First, the choices that patients make each day in managing their diabetes have a greater impact on their outcomes than the decisions made by health care professionals. Second, patients are in control of their self-management behaviors. As health care professionals, we can educate, cajole, and attempt to motivate, but patients have control over the decisions they make once they return to their homes. They can also choose different recommendations to follow each day. Third, the consequences for these decisions accrue first and foremost to patients. Diabetes, including its daily management, belongs to the person with the illness.

INFLUENCES ON BEHAVIOR CHANGE

The level of behavior change required to manage diabetes is difficult for most people. Despite the innate desire that most adults have to be healthy and live a long, independent life, it is often difficult to maintain the behaviors required for a lifetime of self-care. Although most patients want to reach the recommended levels of glycemic control, they also want diabetes to interfere as little as possible with their normal lifestyle and routines.

Diabetes self-management education is essential for behavior change. However, a one-time education program is generally not sufficient to sustain self-care behaviors over a lifetime of diabetes. Making and maintaining behavior changes requires considerable motivation on the part of most patients. It is tempting to try to motivate patients through use of positive or negative reinforcement (e.g., praise, criticism, fear tactics). However, the motivation required to make and sustain behavior changes for chronic illness care is most effective when it comes from within the patient and is directed at changes that are personally valued and meaningful.

Research related to self-determination theory predicts that when patients are given autonomy (a sense of choices and self-initiation) and helped to identify what is important to them and set goals, they are more internally motivated to care for their diabetes than when they are feeling controlled or pressured. In addition, feeling more confident about making and sustaining behavior changes (self-efficacy) and decisional balance (weighing positive and negative effects of behavior change) also influence behavior change. Cultural beliefs and values and family and other social support can also serve as positive or negative influences.

Psychosocial factors can also affect patients' abilities to make and sustain behavior changes. For example, depression is much more common among people with diabetes and can negatively impact self-efficacy and motivation. Most patients, including those with good glycemic control, also indicate that diabetes causes emotional distress and that these concerns are rarely addressed in their interactions with health care professionals. Encouraging patients to talk about these feelings and actively listening to their responses is not only therapeutic but can help uncover issues that may be detrimental to the patients' self-management and quality of life.

For many years, behavior change was synonymous with patient compliance. Health care professionals were viewed as the authorities on diabetes care and patients were expected to adhere or follow their advice. However, patients often resisted professional advice as an encroachment on their autonomy. As a result, many patients jeopardized their physical health to maintain their sense of emotional well-being.

In contrast to this view are more patient-centered or collaborative models of diabetes care. Patients are increasingly recognized as the decision-makers and leaders in their own self-care. This approach is compatible with the Chronic Disease Model for health care delivery, which is based on an active collaboration between patients and providers.

In this model, the role of health care professionals is to provide patients with knowledge and skills for informed decision-making, attempt to understand the patient's perspective about diabetes, acknowledge feelings and cultural and family influences and values, and support the patient's efforts in achieving self-selected diabetes care goals.

STRATEGIES FOR BEHAVIOR CHANGE

Strategies for behavior change are based on autonomy motivation and autonomy support. *Autonomy motivation* is the internal process that drives behavior change. Table 6.1 outlines questions to assess autonomy motivation.

Autonomy support refers to the behaviors that professionals explicitly use to enhance motivation and self-directed behavior change. One of the most powerful strategies that providers can use to provide this type of support is setting goals. Establishing collaborative goals with patients greatly increases the likelihood that patients will be able to achieve those goals.

Table 6.1 Assessing Autonomy Motivation

- What about diabetes is causing you the most anxiety or distress?
- What about this situation needs to change for you to feel better about it?
- What will you gain if you make this change?
- What will you have to give up?
- How will you feel if things do not change?
- On a scale of 1–10, how important is it for you to make a change in this situation?
- What can you do to bring about this change?

Most patients will need assistance in learning to set meaningful, measurable, and realistic goals. Table 6.2 outlines a five-step process for goal-setting that supports collaboration. When setting goals, it is helpful to encourage patients to think of these as experiments, rather than as absolutes that will result in a success or a failure. Beginning the next visit by asking patients about their experiment and what they learned as a result sets the agenda for the rest of the visit and future goal-setting.

SELF-MANAGEMENT SUPPORT

Most studies indicate that sustaining behavioral changes is more difficult than making an initial change. Patients will need ongoing follow-up and support to

Table 6.2 Self-Directed Goal-Setting

Identify the Problem
- What is the most difficult or frustrating part of caring for your diabetes at this time?

Determine Feelings and Their Influence on Behavior
- How do you feel about this issue?
- How are your feelings influencing your behavior?

Set a Long-Term Goal
- What do you want?
- What do you need to do?
- What problems do you expect to encounter?
- What support do you have to overcome these problems?
- Are you willing/able to take action to address these problems?

Make a Plan for a Behavioral Step
- What will you do this week to get started working toward your goal?

Assess the "Experiment"
- How did it work?
- What did you learn?
- What might you do differently next time?

maintain the gains made through a self-management education program or initial goal-setting. This type of support includes

- following up on goals set
- assisting with stress, distress, and coping
- collaborating to solve problems and overcome barriers
- providing information about new or different treatment options
- setting new goals or recommitting to or revising existing goals

REDESIGNING PRACTICE TO SUPPORT BEHAVIOR CHANGE

Most health care delivery systems are designed to provide acute rather than chronic disease care. In recent years, there have been growing pressures on providers to see more and more patients in less time with fewer resources and support staff. There are, however, strategies that providers can use to support behavior change among their patients with diabetes. Table 6.3 outlines health care professional and practice-based strategies that can support effective self-management. Not all of this support needs to be done by clinicians. Nurses or other trained office staff can meet with patients before the visit and assess progress toward goals, establish an agenda for the visit, and set a new goal. Use of other health care professionals outside the practice (certified diabetes educators, dietitians, case mangers), support groups, lay health workers, and community resources can also provide this type of support.

Table 6.3 Provider and Practice-Based Strategies to Support Behavior Change

Provider Strategies
- Stress the importance of the patient's role in daily self-care and decision-making to achieve outcomes.
- Begin each visit with an assessment of the patient's progress toward goals, questions, and concerns.
- Provide information about the costs and benefits of behavioral and therapeutic options.
- Provide information about and referrals to diabetes self-management education programs, support groups, and community resources.

Practice-Based Strategies
- Create a supportive, patient-centered environment.
- Use waiting time to provide information and behavioral support.
- Supplement information provided to patients using technology.
- Incorporate behavioral support into interventions coordinated by nurses, case managers, or other office staff members.
- Replace individual visits with group or cluster visits.
- Assist patients to select an area of behavior change that is supported by all staff members at each visit.

CONCLUSION

Behavior change is a critical aspect of diabetes care that greatly affects patients' outcomes and quality of life. Health care professionals have a significant role to play in supporting behavior changes made by patients to effectively manage their diabetes on a daily basis. They can provide information about diabetes and referrals for diabetes self-management education programs, stress the importance of the patient's role in his or her own outcomes, teach the skills involved in behavior change, set collaborative goals, and provide on-going behavioral support to assist patients to make and sustain these critical changes.

BIBLIOGRAPHY

Anderson BJ, Rubin RR (Eds.): *Practical Psychology for Diabetes Clinicians.* 2nd ed. Alexandria, VA, American Diabetes Association, 2003

Anderson RM, Funnell MM: *The Art of Empowerment: Stories and Strategies for Diabetes Educators.* Alexandria, VA, American Diabetes Association, 2000

Funnell MM, Anderson RM: Changing healthcare systems and office practice to facilitate patient self-management. *Curr Diab Rep* 3:127–133, 2003

Glasgow RE, Davis CL, Funnell MM, Beck A: Implementing practical interventions to support chronic illness self-management. *Jt Comm J Qual Saf* 29:563–574, 2003

Mensing C, Boucher J, Cypress M, Weinger K, Mulcahy K, Barta P, Hosey G, Kopher W, Lasichak A, Lamb B, Mangan M, Norman J, Tanja J, Yauk L, Wisdom K, Adams C: National standards for diabetes self-management education. *Diabetes Care* 27:S143–S150, 2004

Rubin RR, Napora JP: Behavior change. In *A CORE Curriculum for Diabetes Educators.* 5th ed. Vol. 3. Chicago, American Association of Diabetes Educators, 2003, p. 67–96

Index

Index note: Page references with an f or a t indicate a figure or a table on the designated page.

Acanthosis nigricans, diabetes associated with, 2, 11t
Acarbose, 4t, 9–10, 52t, 54–55t, 57
Acesulfame K, 45
Acromegaly, 9t
"Adipokines," 56
Adiponectin, 22
Adipose tissue
  as an endocrine organ, 22
  insulin resistance of tissue of, 19, 20, 24f
Adolescents, managing type 2 diabetes in, 5, 6, 80, 85–86
Adult-onset diabetes, as type 2 diabetes, 6
African-American population
  diabetes screening of, 11t
  incidence of ESRD in, 112
  managing hypertension in, 105
  risk and incidence of diabetes in, 5, 6
Age, incidence of type 2 diabetes with, 5, 6
Alcohol, in diabetic eating plans, 38t, 46
Aldosteronoma, 9t
American Academy of Pediatrics, 85
American Diabetes Association (ADA)
  on aspirin therapy for dyslipidemia, 103
  Clinical Practice Recommendations of, x
  diagnostic and classification criteria of DM, 3

AMP-dependent protein kinase (AMPK), 48
Angiotensin-converting enzyme (ACE) inhibitors, 104–105, 114
Angiotensin-receptor blockers (ARBs), 104, 114
Anti-insulin receptor antibodies, diabetes associated with, 9t
Asian-American population
  diabetes screening in, 11t
  type 2 diabetes in, 6, 19
Aspartame, 45
Aspart insulin, 59, 60t
Aspirin therapy, 103
Atypical antipsychotics, diabetes induced by, 9t
Australia, diabetes in aboriginal populations of, 19
Autoantibodies to insulin (IAAs), 5
Autonomic neuropathy, 118–120
Autonomy motivation, 126–127, 127t
Autonomy support, 126–127, 127t
Average glycated hemoglobin A_{1c} (A1C)
  evaluating treatment efficacy with, 72, 73–74
  treatment target of, 32, 33, 34t, 36, 53

Behavior changes and maintenance of
  assessing autonomy motivation for, 126–127, 127t

Behavior changes and maintenance of (*Continued*)
  cultural beliefs influencing, 126
  decisional balance influences of, 126
  goal-setting for, 127, 127t, 128
  influences on, 125–126
  patient responsibility for, ix, 5, 125
  psychosocial factors affecting, 126
  role of health care professionals and systems in, 128, 128t, 129
  self-efficacy of, 126
β-adrenergic agonists, diabetes induced by, 9t
β-blockers, 104
β-cell dysfunction
  by autoimmune process, 5
  effects of pharmacologic agents on, 56
  in other specific types of diabetes mellitus, 9t
  role in type 2 diabetes, 6, 18, 19, 20, 22–24, 24t
  in type 1 immune-mediated DM, 5
Biguanide, 30, 52t, 53
Blood pressure. *see also* Hypertension
  complications associated with diabetes, 7, 8t, 11t
  management of hypertension in, 103–104, 104t, 105
  treatment target in type 2 diabetes, 34t
Body mass index (BMI)
  in diabetes screening, 11t, 85–86
  influence on degree of insulin resistance, 20–21
  in pre-diabetes, 9
Buyer's Guide to Diabetes Products (ADA), 72
Bypass Angioplasty Revascularization Investigation, 108

Calcium-channel blockers, 104, 114
Carbohydrate intolerance, 3
Carbohydrates
  distribution in daily intake of, 44

  managing blood glucose with, 37–38, 38t, 39, 43–44
Cardiovascular disease
  effects of exercise on markers of, 48–49
  modifying vascular risk factors for, 102–104, 104t, 105–106, 106t, 107
  screening for, 102
  treatment of, 107–108
  trials/studies on, ix, 108
Cardiovascular reflexes, impaired, 119
Carpal tunnel syndrome, 120
Casual plasma glucose concentration, 12t
Central adiposity
  as cardiovascular risk factor, 102
  effects of exercise on, 49
  in metabolic syndrome, 7, 8t
Charcot arthropathy, 114, 118
Chemical-induced diabetes, 9t
Childhood diabetes, 5, 6, 80, 85–86
Chlorpropamide, 52t, 54–55t, 58, 58t
Cholecystokinin (CCK), 23
Cholesterol
  decreased HDL in metabolic syndrome, 7, 8t
  diabetes associated with low HDL levels, 11t
  dietary intake of, 43
  lipid guidelines for children of, 86
  treatment target in type 2 diabetes for, 34t, 38, 38t, 105–106, 106t, 107
Chromosome 7, defect of, 9t
Chromosome 12, defect of, 9t
Chromosome 20, defect of, 9t
Chronic Disease Model, 126
Clozapine, diabetes induced by, 9t
Coagulation abnormalities in metabolic syndrome, 7
Compliance, behavior changes and maintenance of, 31, 124–127, 127t, 128, 128t, 129
Complications associated with diabetes
  diabetic nephropathy as, 3, 33, 112, 112t, 113–114

microvascular and macrovascular, ix, 3, 6, 29, 101–104, 104t, 105–106, 106t, 107–108
myocardial infarction as, 3, 101, 102
neuropathies in, 3, 118–121
peripheral artery disease as, 3
retinopathy in, 3, 33, 108–109, 109t, 110–111, 111t, 112
stroke as, 3
Congenital rubella, diabetes induced by, 9t
Congestive heart failure (CHF), glitazone treatment and, 56
Continuous insulin infusion, 66
Coronary vessel disease, associated with type 2 diabetes, 101–104, 104t, 105–106, 106t, 107–108
Cranial neuropathy, 120
Cushing's syndrome, 9t
Cystic fibrosis, 9t
Cytomegalovirus, diabetes induced by, 9t

Dairy products, saturated fats in, 43
Detemir insulin, 60, 60t
Diabetes Control and Complications Trial (DCCT), 33, 72, 110
Diabetes Forecast, 72
Diabetes mellitus. see also Type 1 diabetes, Type 2 diabetes
as cardiovascular risk factor, 102
clinical classes of, 3–10
diagnosis and classification of, 2, 3–12, 12t, 13, 14t, 15, 15t, 16
risk factors for, 3, 5, 6, 7, 11t, 18–20, 24f
screening for, 2, 10–11, 11t, 85–86
Diabetes Prevention Program (DPP), ix, 3, 7, 9
Diabetic amyotrophy, 120
Diabetic foot problems
causes of, 114–115
nontraumatic amputations related to, 114
prevention of, 115, 115t, 116t, 117f/t
signs and symptoms of, 116t

tendon shortening in, 114
treatment of, 117
Diabetic neuropathies
autonomic neuropathies in, 118–120
diagnosis and treatment of, 120–121
polyneuropathy, 118
Diabetic renal disease
clinical presentation of, 112, 112t, 113
conditions associated with, 113
prevention and treatment of, 113–114
Diabetic retinopathy
evaluating for, 110–111, 111t
incidence and prevalence of, 108
patient education about, 108–109, 109t
prevention of, 110–111, 111t
stages of, 109–110
treatment of, 111–112
Diabetic Retinopathy Study, 110
Diarrhea, diabetic, 119
Diazoxide, diabetes induced by, 9t
Diet. see Nutrition/diet
DIGAMI Study Group, 74
Dilantin, diabetes induced by, 9t
Down's syndrome, diabetes associated with, 9t
Drugs/medications. see also Pharmacologic interventions; *specific medication*
diabetes induced by, 9t
drugs causing hyper/hypoglycemia, 31
toxic effects on renal function by, 113

Early Treatment Diabetic Retinopathy Study, 103, 110
Elderly population, incidence of type 2 diabetes in, 6
End-stage renal disease (ESRD), 112
Entrapment neuropathies, 120
Ethnic/minority populations. see also *specific population*
epidemic incidence of type 2 diabetes in, 5, 6, 11t

Exercise
benefits of, 9, 31, 48–49
effects on pre-diabetes, 9
impact on vascular risk factors,
48–49, 102–103
individualized goals and therapies
for type 2 diabetes, 30, 49
physical activity in U.S. schools, 85
as predictor to weight maintenance,
39, 49
preexercise evaluations and, 50, 50t,
51, 51t
recommended types and duration
of, 49
Exocrine pancreas, diseases of, 9t
Extendin-4, 23

Fasting plasma glucose (FPG), 2
evaluating for pharmacologic interventions, 61–63
in pre-diabetes, 8
as test of choice, 2, 11–12, 12t
Fat cells. *see* Adipose tissue
Fats
effects on lipid levels, 38, 41–42,
42t, 43
fat substitutes in, 45
monounsaturated fats in, 41–42, 42t
saturated fats in, 38, 42–43
trans fatty acids in, 38, 43
Fatty acids, ω-3, 43
Femoral neuropathy, 120
Fenofibrate, 107
Fiber, impact on carbohydrate absorption, 38t, 44
Fibrates, 107
Fibrinolysis, abnormalities in metabolic syndrome, 7
Fibrocalculous pancreatopathy, 8, 9t
Fish oil, 43
Foot problems, diabetic, 114–115,
115t, 116t, 117, 117f/t
Free fatty acids (FFAs)
influence on liver response to
insulin, 21, 24f
in normal secretion of insulin, 22,
24f

Friedreich's ataxia, diabetes associated
with, 9t
Fructose sweetener, 44

Gastric inhibitory peptides (GIP-1 and
GIP-2), 23
Gastrin, 23
Gastroparesis, 119
Gemfibrozil, 107
Genetics
disorders in other specific types of
diabetes, 8, 9t
glucose intolerance as common
denominator in DM, 3
risk factors for type 2 diabetes, 18,
19–20, 24f
"thrifty genes" as risk for diabetes,
19, 24f
Gestational diabetes mellitus (GDM)
clinical characteristics of, 4t, 10, 11
as clinical class of DM, 3
diagnostic criteria for, 12–13, 13t
as risk factor for type 2 diabetes, 7,
10, 11
screening for, 2
Glargine insulin, 60, 60t
Glimepiride, 52t, 54–55t, 58, 58t, 62
"Glinides," 30, 52t, 54–55t, 58t, 59
Glipizide, 52t, 54–55t, 58, 58t, 62
Glucagon-like peptide (GLP)-1, 23
Glucagonoma, 9t
Glucocorticoids, diabetes induced by,
9t
Glucose intolerance
as genetic factor in diabetes, 3
as part of metabolic syndrome, 7, 8t
"Glucose toxicity," 53
α-glucosidase inhibitors, 30, 52, 52t,
54–55t, 57, 62
Glulisine insulin, 59, 60t
Glutamic acid decarboxylase (GAD), 5
Glyburide, 52t, 54–55t, 58, 58t, 59
Glycated hemoglobin. *see* Average gly-
cated hemoglobin A_{1c} (A1C)
Glycemic control
assessing treatment efficacy of,
31–32, 71, 71t, 72–77

impact of exercise on, 48
loss of, 31
optimizing control in type 2 diabetes, 99, 100–101
pharmacologic interventions for, 30–31
pregnancy, before and during, 80, 83
reducing vascular complications with, 99
Glycemic food index/glycemic response, 44

Hands, diabetic neuropathies of, 118, 120–121
HDL cholesterol levels in metabolic syndrome, 7, 8t
Heart Protection Study, 103
Hemochromatosis, 9t
Hepatic nuclear factor (HNF), defects of, 9t
Hispanic/Latino population
diabetes screening in, 11t
incidence of ESRD in, 112
prevalence of metabolic syndrome in, 7
risk and incidence of diabetes in, 5, 6, 19
HMG CoA-reductase inhibitors (statins), 106–107
Hospitalization, managing diabetes during, 80–81, 88–89, 89t
Human leukocyte antigen (HLA), 5
Huntington's chorea, diabetes associated with, 9t
Hyperglycemia, ix, 3
Hyperinsulinemia, 7
Hyperosmolar hyperglycemic state (HHS)
electrolyte deficits of, 92–94
pathophysiology of, 81, 91
treatments of, 92–94
Hyperosmolar nonketotic coma (HHNC), 91
Hyperproinsulinemia, 9t
Hypertension
diabetes associated with, 11t

management of, 103–104, 104t, 105
in metabolic syndrome, 7, 8t
nephropathy associated with, 113
Hyperthyroidism, 9t
Hyperuricemia, in metabolic syndrome, 7
Hypoglycemia
as complications of sulfonylurea treatment, 57–58
exercise-induced, 49, 50

Immune-mediated diabetes, uncommon forms of, 9t
Impaired fasting glucose (IFG), 2, 3
Impaired glucose tolerance (IGT), ix, 2, 3, 7, 11t
Incretin hormone, 23
India, incidence of type 2 diabetes in, 19
Indinavir, diabetes induced by, 9t
Infections, diabetes induced by, 9t
Inflammation, role in metabolic syndrome, 7, 8t
Inpatient hospitalization, managing diabetes during, 88–89, 89t
Insulin
action of, 61
autoantibodies (IAAs), 5
β-cell function and, 31
factors modulating secretion of, 18, 23, 24f
genetic defects in, 9t
hyperinsulinemia in, 7
impact of exercise on sensitivity to, ix, 48
insulin pump therapy of, 66–67
intensive/intravenous insulin therapy, 88–89, 89t
intermediate-acting, 60t
long-acting, 60t
mixtures, 60, 60t, 61
multiple daily injection (MDI) regimen, 66
mutant insulins in, 9t
regimens in long-term type 2 diabetes, 65, 68t, 69

Insulin (*Continued*)
  secretion defects with type 2 dia-
    betes, 22–23
  short-acting, 60t
  starting therapy with, 4t, 5, 31,
    54–55t, 59–60, 60t, 61, 63–65,
    65t, 66–67
  timing of SMBG with regimen of,
    65, 65t, 66, 67, 75
Insulin-dependent diabetes mellitus
    (IDDM). *see* Type 1 diabetes
Insulin-promoter factor-1, defect of,
    9t
Insulin resistance syndrome
  defined, 20
  mechanisms of, 20–22, 24f
  as part of metabolic syndrome, 7, 8t
  postreceptor abnormalities role in,
    21
  tissue sites of, 18, 20, 24f
  in type 2 diabetes, 7, 19, 24f
α-Interferon, diabetes induced by, 9t
Interleukin (IL)-6, 22
Intra-abdominal fat, insulin resistance
    with, 7, 8t, 21, 49, 102
Islet cell autoantibodies (ICAs), 5

Juvenile-onset diabetes. *see* Type 1
    diabetes

Ketoacidosis in type 2 diabetes, 6
Klinefelter's syndrome, diabetes asso-
    ciated with, 9t
Kumamoto study, 74, 100, 110

Lactic acidosis, risk of, 53
Latent autoimmune diabetes of aging
    (LADA), in pathogenesis of
    DM, 5
Laurence-Moon-Biedl syndrome, dia-
    betes associated with, 9t
Lente insulin, 60t
Leprechaunism, 9t
Leptin, 22
Lifestyle

  modifying vascular risk factors in,
    102–104, 104t, 105–106, 106t,
    107
  sedentary lifestyle linked with type 2
    diabetes, 5, 7
  type 2 diabetes therapies with
    changes in, 54–55t
Lipids
  dyslipidemia associated with type 2
    diabetes, 41, 105–106, 106t, 107
  effects of fats on levels of, 38, 41–42,
    42t, 43
  effects of glitazones on levels of,
    56–57
  guidelines for pediatric levels of, 86
Lipoatrophic diabetes, 9t
Lipodystrophy, 22
Lispro insulin, 59, 60t
Liver, insulin resistance of tissue of,
    19, 20, 24f
Lumbosacral plexus neuropathies, 120

Macrovascular complications
  associated with type 2 diabetes,
    101–104, 104t, 105–106, 106t,
    107–108
  myocardial infarction as, 3
  peripheral artery disease as, 3
  prevention of, 29
  stroke as, 3
"Malnutrition-related diabetes." *see*
    Fibrocalculous pancreatopathy
Mannitol sweetener, 44, 45
Maturity-onset diabetes of the young
    (MODY)
  classification of, 7–8, 9t, 15
  genetic aberrations in, 19, 24f
Medical nutrition therapy in type 2
    diabetes. *see also* Nutrition/diet
approaches to weight reduction in,
    38t, 39–40
assessing weight and BMI for,
    37–38, 38t, 39–40
assessment and health care team in,
    36
goals of, 36

Medications. *see* Drugs/medications; Pharmacologic interventions; *specific medication*

Metabolic syndrome, criteria for diagnosis of, 7, 8t

Metformin
  beginning a treatment with, ix, 33, 52, 52t, 53, 54–55t, 61, 62
  effects on pre-diabetes, 4t, 9
  for type 2 diabetes in children, 80

Microalbuminuria, in metabolic syndrome, 7, 8t

Microvascular complications with diabetes
  diabetic retinopathy in, 3, 33, 103, 109–112
  neuropathies in, ix, 3, 6, 29, 33, 118–120
  prevention of, 29

Miglitol, 52t, 54–55t, 57

Mitochondrial DNA, defects of, 9t

Monounsaturated fats, 41–42, 42t

Muscle
  exercise and oxidative capacity of, 48
  insulin resistance of tissue of, 19, 20–21, 24f

Mutant insulins, 9t

Myocardial infarction, as macrovascular complication of DM, ix, 3, 101, 102

Myotonic dystrophy, diabetes associated with, 9t

Nateglinide, 52t, 53, 54–55t, 58t, 59, 62

National Cholesterol Education Program Adult Treatment Panel III (NCEP-ATP III)
  criteria for diagnosis of metabolic syndrome by, 7, 8t
  on management of dyslipidemia, 105–106, 106t, 107

National Cholesterol Education Program (NCEP), 86, 105–106

National Diabetes Data Group, 3

National Health and Nutrition Examination Survey, 7–8

National Standards for Diabetes Self-Management Education, 34

National Weight Control Registry, 49

Native American population
  diabetes screening of, 11t
  incidence of ESRD in, 112
  risk and incidence of diabetes in, 5, 6, 19

Nelfinavir, diabetes induced by, 9t

Neotame, 45

Nephropathy, diabetic, 3, 33, 112, 112t, 113–114

Neuroarthropathy, 114–115

NeuroD1/BETA2, defect of, 9t

Neurogenic bladder, 113, 119

Neuropathies, diabetic, 3, 33, 118–121

Nicotinic acid, 9t, 107

Nonalcoholic fatty liver disease, diabetes associated with, 7

Non-insulin-dependent diabetes mellitus (NIDDM), 6

Nonsulfonylurea, 52t, 53, 54–55t

Norwegian timolol study, 108

NPH, 60, 60t

Nutrition/diet. *see also* Medical nutrition therapy in type 2 diabetes
  carbohydrate distribution in daily intake of, 30
  "dieting," psychological and physiological impact of, 39
  effects on pre-diabetes, 9
  fat intake and type 2 diabetes, 38t, 41–42, 42t, 43
  glycemic food index/glycemic response in, 44
  modifying vascular risk factors with, 103
  obstacles to dietary adherence of, 37t
  protein intake in type 2 diabetes, 38t, 40–41
  recommended goals and principles of, 38t
  role in developing type 2 diabetes, 6, 20, 24f
  serving sizes for each food group, 43
  therapies for type 2 diabetes, 29–30
  vitamins and minerals in, 38t, 45–46

Obesity
β-cell number associated with, 22, 24f
central adiposity in, 7, 8t, 21, 49, 102
effects of Westernized diet on, 6
increase in pediatric patients, ix, 85
screening for diabetes with, 2, 10–11, 11t, 85–86
visceral obesity as risk factor, 7
weight loss therapies for, 29
Olanzapine, diabetes induced by, 9t
Olestra, 45
Oral antidiabetic agents
biguanide/metformin in, ix, 4t, 9, 30, 33, 52, 52t, 53, 54–55t, 61, 62, 80
α-glucosidase inhibitors in, 30, 52, 52t, 54–55t, 62
thiazolidinediones in, 10, 30, 52, 52t, 53, 54–55t, 56–57, 61, 62
Oral glucose tolerance test (OGTT), in diagnosis of diabetes, 2, 8, 11–12, 12t, 13, 13t
Orlistat, 10
Orthostatic hypotension, 119
Other specific types of diabetes
clinical characteristics of, 4t
as clinical class of DM, 3, 4, 5
criteria and correct diagnosis of, 7–8, 9t

Pacific Islander population
diabetes screening of, 11t
risk and incidence of diabetes in, 6, 19
Pancreatectomy, diabetes induced by, 9t
Pancreatitis, diabetes induced by, 9t
Pathogenesis of type 2 diabetes, 18–24, 24f
Patient education
about diabetic retinopathy, 109t
on diabetic foot problems, 115, 115t, 116t, 117f/t
on diabetic nephropathy, 3, 33, 112, 112t, 113

on proper self-monitoring methods, 74–77
on successful changes for self-care, ix, 29, 125–127, 127t, 128, 128t, 129
Pediatrics
differentiating type 1 and type 2 diabetes in, 85
managing type 2 diabetes in, 80, 85–86
Pentamidine, diabetes induced by, 9t
Peripheral artery disease, associated with DM, 3
Pharmacologic interventions
as adjunct therapy, 30
by augmenting the supply of insulin, 52t, 54–55t, 57–58, 58t, 59
beginning a treatment with, 61–63
for control of dyslipidemia, 106–107
drugs causing hyper/hypo-glycemia, 31
by enhancing the effectiveness of insulin, 52, 52t, 53, 54–55t, 56–57
for hypertension, 104, 104t, 105
insulin therapy without oral agents, 64–65, 65t, 66–67
long-term combinations of oral with insulin, 67–68, 68t, 69
in managing high-risk obesity, 40
oral antidiabetic agents in, ix, 4t, 30, 33, 52, 52t, 53, 54–55t, 61, 62, 80
primary and secondary failure of, 63
starting insulin therapy, 63–65, 65t, 66–67
Pheochromocytoma, 9t
Phosphorylations, disorders with insulin resistance, 21
Physician's Health Study, 103
Pioglitazone, 10, 52t, 54–55t, 57
Polycystic ovary syndrome (PCOS), diabetes associated with, 2, 7, 11t, 85
Polydipsia, 6
Polyneuropathy, 118
Polyphagia, 6
Polyuria, 6

Porphyria, diabetes associated with, 9t
Prader-Willi syndrome, diabetes associated with, 9t
Pre-diabetes
    ADA recommendation of lifestyle changes with, 9, 10
    clinical characteristics of, 3, 4t
    diagnostic criteria for, 8, 12
Pregnancy. *see also* Gestational diabetes mellitus (GDM)
    managing type 2 diabetes before and during, 80, 83
    maternal and fetal risks with, 83
Primary failure of treatment, 63
Protease inhibitors, diabetes induced by, 9t
Protein
    effects on renal insufficiency, 41
    recommended intake in type 2 diabetes, 38t, 40–41

Quetiapine, diabetes induced by, 9t

Rabson-Mendenhall syndrome, 9t
Reaven, Gerald M., 7
Regular insulin, 60t
Renal disease
    diabetic renal disease in, 112, 112t, 113–114
    end stage renal disease (ESRD), 112
    modifying protein intake for, 40–41
Repaglinide, 52t, 53, 54–55t, 58t, 59
Resistin, 22
Retinopathy, diabetic, 3, 33, 103, 109, 109t, 110–112
Reye's syndrome, 103
Risperidone, diabetes induced by, 9t
Ritonavir, diabetes induced by, 9t
Rosiglitazone, 10, 52t, 54–55t, 56

Saccharin, 45
Saquinavir, diabetes induced by, 9t
Saturated fats, 42–43
Screening for diabetes, 2, 10–11, 11t, 85–86

Secondary failure of treatment, 63
Secretin, 23
Sedentary lifestyle, as risk factor for type 2 diabetes, ix, 19, 20, 24f, 48–49
Self-care, behavior changes for, 125–127, 127t, 128, 128t, 129
Self-determination theory, 126
Self-monitoring of blood glucose (SMBG)
    assessing treatment efficacy with, 71, 71t, 72–76
    monitoring pharmacologic interventions with, 31, 32, 36, 40, 65, 65t
Semmes-Weinstein monofilament examination, 115, 117f/t
Sexual dysfunction in men, 120
Smoking, cardiovascular risks associated with, 107
Somatostatinoma, 9t
Sorbitol sweetener, 44, 45
Statins, 106–107
Steno-2 Study, 33
"Stiff-man" syndrome, diabetes associated with, 9t
Stroke, as macrovascular complication of DM, 3
Studies. *see* Trials/studies
Sucralose, 45
Sucrose (table sugar), 44
Sugar/sugar substitutes, 38t, 44–45
Sulfonylurea receptor (SUR), 57, 59
Sulfonylureas, 30, 33, 52t, 53, 54–55t, 57–58, 58t, 59, 62
Surgeon General's Report on Physical Activity and Health, 49
Surgery, managing diabetes during, 88–89, 89t
Sweeteners, 38t, 44–45

Television viewing, correlation with weight problems, 85
Thiazide, diabetes induced by, 9t
Thiazolidinediones, 10, 30, 52, 52t, 53, 54–55t, 56–57, 61, 62
"Thrifty genes," 19, 24f

Thyroid hormone, diabetes induced by, 9t
Tolazamide, 52t, 54–55t, 58, 58t
Tolbutamide, 52t, 54–55t, 58, 58t
Trans fatty acids, 38, 43
Treat-to-Target Trial, 65, 67
Trials/studies
  on benefits of exercise, 48, 49
  Bypass Angioplasty Revascularization Investigation in, 108
  cardiovascular intervention trials in, ix, 108
  Diabetes Control and Complications Trial (DCCT) in, 33, 72, 110
  Diabetes Prevention Program (DPP) in, ix, 3, 7, 9
  Diabetic Retinopathy Study in, 110
  DIGAMI Study in, 74
  Early Treatment Diabetic Retinopathy Study in, 103, 110
  Heart Protection Study in, 103
  Kumamoto study in, 74, 100, 110
  Norwegian timolol study in, 108
  Physician's Health Study in, 103
  Steno-2 Study in, 33
  Treat-to-Target Trial in, 65, 67
  United Kingdom Prospective Diabetes Study (UKPDS) in, ix, 33, 61, 63, 72, 100–101, 103, 110
  VA-HIT study in, 107
  on vitamin and minerals, 45–46
  Wisconsin Epidemiologic Study of Diabetic Retinopathy in, 110
Triglyceride levels
  accumulations of intracellular stores of, 21–22, 24f
  diabetes associated with, 11t
  effects of glitazones on levels of, 56–57
  managing dyslipidemia in type 2 diabetes in, 105–106, 106t, 107
  in metabolic syndrome, 7, 8t
  treatment target of, 34t, 49
Troglitazone, reducing risk of developing diabetes with, 10
Truncal radiculopathy, 120
Tumor necrosis factor (TNF)-α, 22

Type A insulin resistance, 9t
Type 1 diabetes
  autoimmune type, 4, 5
  clinical characteristics of, 4t, 5
  as clinical class of DM, 3
  developing ketoacidosis with, 2
  diagnostic criteria for, 5, 11–12, 12t
  idiopathic class of, 5
  immune-mediated class of, 5
  as insulin deficiency, 2
  prevalence and incidence of, 5
  specific markers of, 15
Type 2 diabetes
  assessing treatment efficacy of, 31–32, 71, 71t, 72–77
  clinical characteristics of, 3, 4t, 6
  commonly associated with obesity, 2, 6, 7, 10–11, 11t, 85–86
  defined, 19
  diagnostic criteria for, 11–12, 12t
  dual defects of, 23–24, 24f
  epidemic incidence of, ix, 6
  etiology of, 6, 7
  gestational diabetes mellitus (GDM) and, 2
  heterogeneous nature of, 36
  individualized therapies in, 29
  insulin resistance with, 19, 24f
  medical nutrition therapy for, 29, 36, 37–38, 38t, 39–40
  metabolic targets and goals of, ix, 29, 33–34, 34t
  pharmacologic therapy for, 29
  physical activity goals for, 29
  populations affected, 5, 6, 11t
  progression of disease of, 31
  risk factors for, 2, 7, 18, 19–20, 24f, 48–49
  "silent" onset of, 99
  treatment goals of, 29

Ulnar neuropathy, 120
Ultralente insulin, 60t
United Kingdom Prospective Diabetes Study (UKPDS), ix, 33, 61, 63, 72, 100–101, 103, 110

United States Dietary Guidelines, 37, 39

United States Food and Drug Administration (FDA), 59, 86

Upper limb mononeuropathies, 120

Urinary tract infection (UTI), 113

Urine glucose measurements, 76

Urine ketone measurement, 76

USDA Food Guide Pyramid, 41, 43

Vacor, diabetes induced by, 9t

VA-HIT study, 107

Vascular disease, as complication of diabetes, ix, 11t, 100t, 101–104, 104t, 105–106, 106t, 107–108

Vasoactive intestinal polypeptide (VIP), 23

Visceral obesity as risk factor, 7

Weight
approaches to reduction of, 6, 9, 38t, 39–40, 42

impact of exercise on, 49

incidence of regaining lost weight, 39, 40

in metabolic syndrome, 7, 8t

normal weight and type 2 diabetes, 37–39

surgical interventions for loss of, 40

visceral obesity as risk factor, 7

Wisconsin Epidemiologic Study of Diabetic Retinopathy, 110

Wolfram's syndrome, diabetes associated with, 9t

World Health Organization (WHO)
criteria for diagnosis of metabolic syndrome by, 7, 8t

on incidence of type 2 diabetes, 6

on proper performance of OGTT, 12, 12t

Youth, managing type 2 diabetes in, 80

About the American Diabetes Association

The American Diabetes Association is the nation's leading voluntary health organization supporting diabetes research, information, and advocacy. Its mission is to prevent and cure diabetes and to improve the lives of all people affected by diabetes. The American Diabetes Association is the leading publisher of comprehensive diabetes information. Its huge library of practical and authoritative books for people with diabetes covers every aspect of self-care—cooking and nutrition, fitness, weight control, medications, complications, emotional issues, and general self-care.

To order American Diabetes Association books: Call 1-800-232-6733. Or log on to http://store.diabetes.org

To join the American Diabetes Association: Call 1-800-806-7801. www.diabetes.org/membership

For more information about diabetes or ADA programs and services: Call 1-800-342-2383. E-mail: Customerservice@diabetes.org or log on to www.diabetes.org

To locate an ADA/NCQA Recognized Provider of quality diabetes care in your area: www.ncqa.org/dprp

To find an ADA Recognized Education Program in your area: Call 1-888-232-0822. www.diabetes.org/recognition/education.asp

To join the fight to increase funding for diabetes research, end discrimination, and improve insurance coverage: Call 1-800-342-2383. www.diabetes.org/advocacy

To find out how you can get involved with the programs in your community: Call 1-800-342-2383. See below for program Web addresses.

- *American Diabetes Month:* Educational activities aimed at those diagnosed with diabetes—month of November. www.diabetes.org/ADM
- *American Diabetes Alert:* Annual public awareness campaign to find the undiagnosed—held the fourth Tuesday in March. www.diabetes.org/alert
- *The Diabetes Assistance & Resources Program (DAR):* Diabetes awareness program targeted to the Latino community. www.diabetes.org/DAR
- *African American Program:* Diabetes awareness program targeted to the African American community. www.diabetes.org/africanamerican
- *Awakening the Spirit: Pathways to Diabetes Prevention & Control:* Diabetes awareness program targeted to the Native American community. www.diabetes.org/awakening

To find out about an important research project regarding type 2 diabetes: www.diabetes.org/ada/research.asp

To obtain information on making a planned gift or charitable bequest: Call 1-888-700-7029. www.diabetes.org/ada/plan.asp

To make a donation or memorial contribution: Call 1-800-342-2383. www.diabetes.org/ada/cont.asp